"Social prescribing is critical to addressing the health of all patients. Traditional medicine covers at best 20% of their needs, and has significant side effects and risks. This book explores how developing communities facilitates lifestyle changes to improve population health."

—**Sir Sam Everington**, *GP, Bromley By Bow Centre.*


"Simon Lennane's book is a treasury of resources of the profound effect of community building on healthcare and beyond, to the future of our planet. The magic of communities has the potential to transform our world and *Creating Community Health* shows how this can be done."

—**Dr Julian Abel**, *Director of Compassionate Communities UK and co-author of 'The Compassion Project'.*

# Creating Community Health

This important book explores how community-based interventions can bridge the gap between health services and the voluntary sector to create more sustainable, healthy communities.

Moving beyond a technologically driven, medicalised approach to healthcare, the book shows how social prescribing can provide a direct pathway to improving community health, embracing connection and challenging inequality. Written by a practicing GP, and illustrated through practical guidance, it demonstrates how this can offer a cost-effective, preventative means to improving health outcomes, enabling communities to be more resilient when confronting major issues such as climate change or pandemics.

Building to a case study of how these methods were used in one town, Ross-on-Wye, the book will be invaluable reading for those working in healthcare, public health, local authorities, and the voluntary sector, as well as students and researchers interested in these areas.

**Dr Simon Lennane** has been a GP in Ross-on-Wye for twenty years. Simon was Clinical Director of the local Primary Care Network during the pandemic, responsible for urgent care and vaccination clinics, and was also clinical lead for mental health commissioning. Simon published research into ethnicity and deaths of healthcare workers from COVID-19. He has long been involved with community development in the town, and was a founder trustee of Ross Community Development Trust, which supports the local voluntary sector.

Twitter: @SimonLennane. Mastodon: @SimonLennane@mas.to

# Creating Community Health

Interventions for Sustainable Healthcare

**Simon Lennane**

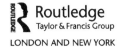 Routledge
Taylor & Francis Group

LONDON AND NEW YORK

Cover credit: © Getty Images

First published 2023
by Routledge
4 Park Square, Milton Park, Abingdon, Oxon OX14 4RN

and by Routledge
605 Third Avenue, New York, NY 10158

*Routledge is an imprint of the Taylor & Francis Group, an informa business*

© 2023 Simon Lennane

*British Library Cataloguing-in-Publication Data*
A catalogue record for this book is available from the British Library

ISBN: 978-1-032-49004-5 (hbk)
ISBN: 978-1-032-14097-1 (pbk)
ISBN: 978-1-003-39178-4 (ebk)

DOI: 10.4324/9781003391784

Typeset in Times New Roman
by SPi Technologies India Pvt Ltd (Straive)

This book is dedicated to all those who take part.

# Contents

# Figures

# Tables

# Foreword

by *Cormac Russell*

This book reveals the potential for health beyond healthcare.

While essential to our health and wellbeing, our healthcare systems have reached the limits of their health-producing and sickness-preventing capacities. The doctor cannot do it all, and the hospital can only patch us up.

Much like the blueprint of the butterfly is encoded within imaginal cells, hidden deep behind the seemingly catastrophic collapse of the caterpillar, so too, in these pages are the imaginal cells of a healthy society and functioning healthcare systems. Just as imaginal cells inside a caterpillar are set apart from other cells because they carry a unique understanding that in the future, the caterpillar will turn into a butterfly, this book is set apart from others because its pages carry a unique set of insights about the necessary metamorphosis that our healthcare systems must go through. Dr Simon Lennane, the author of this important and compelling book, is an active thought leader in the domain of community health and a GP who understands communities' complex nature and possibilities. He also understands the limits of the biomedical model.

If we carefully follow Simon's coordinates, iatrogenic interventions will be lowered, and health supports will result in more meaningful and enduring impacts across populations. But that is not the actual prize to be discovered in this book. These chapters have a unique offering in that they carry a deep understanding that in the future, our health will be made manifest beyond the real estate of health systems; the evidence of their impacts will be found not in our hospitals or clinics but in our communities and local economies. I would contend that it was ever thus, because beyond the limits of medicine, health is contingent on the depth and quality of social connectedness and principles of social justice. The most pressing need is not more hospital beds but more hospitable communities. Yet the national conversation is stuck on the former at the latter's expense.

Raymond Williams cautions that 'To be truly radical is to make hope possible rather than despair convincing'. By that definition, we can say Simon is a true radical in that he deftly calls attention to the root of what is ailing us and our natural world. And he does so in an open-hearted way. His diagnoses and ultimate prognoses lay neither blame nor shame on our health institutions or those that use them. He is neither an apologist nor an abolitionist. If we were to categorise him at all, we would have to invent a new term, which captures the fact that he has gone beyond well-rehearsed public narratives that call for deeper institutional reforms, or behaviour and lifestyle change 'scripts' that all too often gaslight people living in economic poverty. One might say he is a 'metamorphosist', in that he helps us to see that an alternative and preferred future for health and care lies beyond the moribund discussions about reform and behaviour change and is to be found in the natural messiness of regular communities. He calls on fellow healers to commit to a much-needed metamorphosis of the healthcare system, which will ultimately relocate some of the authority and resources for health creation back to the very people it serves and their collective capacities.

The metamorphosis described thoroughly throughout this book is a sobering yet hopeful reminder that sustainable progress is contingent on understanding the limits of institutional monopolies and the potential of whole community health creation.

Echoing *The Marmot Review* and its '10 Years On' report, Dr Lennane argues that individual and collective choice and control in our (shared) lives and circumstances are essential drivers for health and wellbeing. The preponderance of national and international evidence confirms his assertion. The World Happiness Report, for example, notes that having the freedom to make life choices is one of the six factors that explain the variation in national wellbeing between countries. What is distinctive about this book, though, is the nuance of his argument; he understands the importance of communities of place and rightly views them as holistic and complex systems in their own right; for him, it takes a village to co-create health.

While robustly advocating for social protections and mounting a full-blooded critique of neoliberal policies, he does not fall foul of the assumption that institutions have a monopoly on producing our social and economic welfare. For him, institutions are, at best, an extension of community power; at worst, they have the potential to do significant harm to community autonomy and collective efficacy. Speaking directly to professionals working in citizen space, he reminds us that there are two tools for health: one is institutions, the other is ground-up community development. Dr Lennane elegantly occupies the gap between healthcare systems and the health-producing capacities of citizens and their associations. He has the credibility to simultaneously and compassionately challenge medical overreach while authenticating and cheering on community health creation.

Taking a community-centred approach to health, as advocated for in this book, promises the following outcomes:

- People can expect to live well together and care for each other, themselves, their environment and the economy, with affordable, accessible services close at hand to supplement their capacities.
- Local food production and food sovereignty will be enhanced and accordingly increase public health, not private wealth, as is currently the case in the UK.

- Caring will become more observable at a cultural level, and the impacts on subjective well-being will commensurately be improved.
- Ameliorative allopathic and transactional, instrumental approaches will be supplanted by salutogenic and empathic community development practices promoting individual and collective choice and control.
- Health will no longer be about the benevolence of 'doctors and health-care allies' and 'patients as passive beneficiaries'. Instead, it will be grounded in community power and changes in the social order so that all can participate in society through valued social roles and with a genuine sense of belonging.
- Health and care will grow because people regularly work and play together.
- There will be a more significant commitment to nurturing health and wellbeing within hyperlocal places, such as neighbourhoods, in effect, recognising the neighbourhood as a primary unit of health.
- There will be a commitment to place-based community-building practices in recognition that people in small communities care more about each other's well-being than people on the other side of the country and because there is no way to change the Country's Health Inequalities all at once.

The healthcare system and the health-creating capacities of local communities are separate wings, learning to be in right relationship with each other; this book shows us how to achieve this essential butterfly effect.

**Cormac Russell** is the author of several books including *Rekindling Democracy* and coauthor of *The Connected Community*.

# Preface

This book explores how the social and physical environments we live in affect our health, and how developing community improves our wellbeing. It explores concepts of community, what health is, how our society influences it and how we have organised ourselves to respond. Demedicalising health, and the evidence for activity lead on to the social infrastructure supporting communities and how this can be nourished. Recognising the effects that COVID-19, climate change and our politics are having on our collective health, developing community offers a way to regain control of our health and wellbeing.

The balance between individual and collective is a constant presence. The same themes keep arising; institutional overreach, which disempowers citizens; how demedicalising improves our health; and the drift from collective to individual responsibility. Healthcare is quick to colonise other provision; this book hopes to explore the territory without appropriating it.

Moving quickly across a wide area means hurrying past interesting areas, leaving only markers for those who want to know more. As such, this book is heavily referenced, providing springboards to other resources. This is the butterfly approach of the generalist, connecting and cross-pollinating. Names closely associated with a concept are given in brackets where it adds context.

Where the impact of COVID-19 has made the most recent data unrepresentative, data from before the pandemic have been used. Throughout the book million may be shortened to mn, similar to bn for billion. This helps users of screen readers, which interpret the letter m to represent metres.

As befits a transition economy, costs are outlined in terms of carbon budget where available as well as sterling. A thousand kilograms (kg) is a tonne (t). Continuing to multiply this by a thousand gives a kilotonne (Kt), a megatonne (Mt) and a gigatonne (Gt). The impact of greenhouse gases is sometimes represented in terms of equivalent tonnes of carbon dioxide, tCO2e.

This book was written using open source software (OpenOffice, Zotero, Manjaro Linux). Illustrations were created in Rstudio. Notes, links, additional material and accompanying resources are available at www. communityhealth.uk

# Introduction

Modern medicine is amazing. There have been huge strides in surgery and therapeutics over recent decades. The sharp end of healthcare is very good at managing disease. Very few generations have had the privilege of living in a time of safe anaesthesia and truly life-saving treatments.

Access to medical care is a fundamental human right, but medical care is not the same as health. And while we are living longer than ever before, increases in life expectancy are slowing. The average improvement in life expectancy in the UK has fallen (Figure I.1) to the lowest sustained level in over a century.

This is happening because healthcare is not addressing the other things that influence our health. The way in which we live our lives, our society and economy, the people we spend time with and the environment around us all determine our health far more than the healthcare available to us.

The boundaries of healthcare are ever shifting, but medicine still has little influence over these wider determinants of our health. Healthcare can itself cause harm by professionalising responses and lessening autonomy. Commercial and political pressures on health provision represent the needs of institutions rather than patients. Healthcare becomes an expensive, reactive, technological resource, to which we hand over responsibility for our health.

How much medicine do we need to be healthy? As medicine becomes more intensive, the benefits reduce. That is to say, the health improvements from increasing expenditure become less as spending increases, eventually reaching a limit of optimal effectiveness.

Improving health means instead addressing the causes of poor health, which mostly relate to the way our societies are structured. Our jobs, connections, resources and surroundings all contribute to our health and resilience. Problems with these manifest in poorer health; loneliness, poverty, inequality, trauma, racism and other forms of marginalisation are very bad for us.

By any measure, our current system is damaging; the health impacts of our politics have never been more visible. Austerity policies are estimated to have caused a third of a million excess deaths in the United Kingdom.[1] The UK's poor Covid response contributed to 169,000 excess deaths within two years.[2]

DOI: 10.4324/9781003391784-1

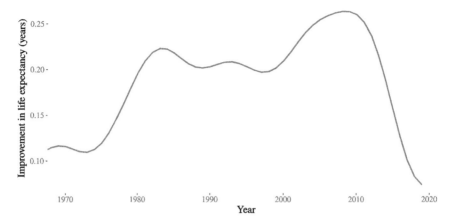

*Figure I.1* Life expectancy change, UK.

Roser M, Ortiz-Ospina E, Ritchie H. Life Expectancy. *Our World Data.*

The gap between rich and poor has never been higher, and COVID-19 has shown how inequality and discrimination still influence the outcomes of a new illness.

Our unsustainable way of life is taking a huge toll on our health. Dependence on fossil fuels is choking us and the planet. Extractive economic systems pollute the air we breathe and water we drink. The growing climate and ecological emergency will put unprecedented stresses on resources, leading to increased migration and conflict. We urgently need to take action to prevent our planet from becoming uninhabitable.

Neoliberalism has normalised inequality and dysfunctional governance. Extractive markets thrive on chaos, but leave economies isolated and fragile. Client media block challenges to power structures. Powerlessness in the face of corruption leads to social breakdown, a dysfunctional society unable to create change effectively enough to survive the challenges ahead. Outsourcing our problems to professionals and politicians has not worked.

Our health systems are ill-equipped to deal with the sociosomatic fallout of a troubled society. Diseases of despair such as alcoholism, suicide and opioid misuse are rooted in social dysfunction. Distress is medicalised while the causes go untreated. Services struggle with the consequences, without the ability to address them. Health services are set up to pull people out of the water, rather than going upstream to stop them falling in. This view presupposes some of us are on the land, but in fact, our health is on a continuum, and we are all in the river. We need to know how to swim.[3]

There is much we can do ourselves and in common with the people around us. Active travel decarbonises our transport and is good for us. Building connections increases our social capital and wellbeing. Our civic environment can do much to support health through access to greenspace, design and a social infrastructure which is health-enabling by default. Sustainable policy is based on transparency, accountability and subsidiarity.

Our social safety net protects us. Made from the ties between people, more connections form a safer net with fewer holes. Crises such as pandemics or extreme weather make the things people do to help each other more visible, creating a collective sense of empowerment and achievement from this mutual support. Volunteering is good for us and our health, participation improving our sense of integration and community cohesion.

Institutions help by supporting while retreating, serving while walking backwards.[4] Providing an infrastructure to support community development enables this without being directive. Connecting people with their communities is an effective health intervention, but involving healthcare medicalises this process. Access to signposting and advice services is helpful to all who work with people. An inclusive society will not need social prescribers.

Making the benefits of community more widely available is effective, but signposting services still need somewhere to signpost to. Developing community capacity helps activity to flourish, creating social capital and improving our health. Communities take control back through participation and empowerment. Individual and community empowerment increases as we join with others to reclaim our influence.

## Notes

Links and additional resources for this chapter can be found at www.communityhealth. uk/introduction

1 Walsh D, Dundas R, McCartney G, Gibson M, Seaman R. Bearing the burden of austerity: how do changing mortality rates in the UK compare between men and women? *J Epidemiol Community Health*. Published online October 4, 2022. doi:10.1136/jech-2022-219645.
2 Wang H, Paulson KR, Pease SA, et al. Estimating excess mortality due to the COVID-19 pandemic: a systematic analysis of COVID-19-related mortality, 2020–21. *The Lancet*. 2022;399(10334):1513–1536. doi:10.1016/S0140-6736(21) 02796-3.
3 Antonovsky A. The salutogenic model as a theory to guide health promotion. *Health Promot Int*. 1996;11(1):11–18. doi:10.1093/heapro/11.1.11.
4 Russell C. *Rekindling Democracy: A Professional's Guide to Working in Citizen Space*. Cascade Books; 2020.

# 1 Community health

Communities are rich, vibrant entities at the heart of our lives. Every community is unique, but the interconnections are the same. Communities exist and interact across locations, interests and experiences. The social cohesion communities bring is a public good, with great benefits to our health. There are ways to encourage the development of communities which enhance the health benefits, providing an effective way to improve population health. Exploring the ways in which people come together allows us to recognise and nurture those things that promote community. This involves working across statutory and voluntary sectors. Understanding common goals and barriers is necessary for these cross-sectoral projects to progress.

The overlap between health and community is well studied, though not currently well integrated within healthcare practice. As a result, patients miss out on effective community-based interventions which reduce costs and demedicalise into a wider associational life. Community health comes from facilitating links into a healthier wider community. Recognising this as a distinct approach within population-based health improvement is an important step towards providing support. The World Health Organisation (WHO) calls community health 'the maintenance and improvement of the health of all the people through collective or social actions'.[1] Community health is, most simply, the role of communities in keeping us healthy.

While the health benefit from community traditionally falls within the field of public health, it is common land, held for the benefit of all and with all responsible for upkeep. Those who work with communities need to recognise the potential effects of their activities on the health of those they serve. Understanding how communities are bound together lets us develop those aspects which are health enabling.

## What is community?

A community is a group joined by common interest or experience. This will often include a geographic element, although increasingly the ability to maintain connections virtually makes other forms of community feasible. The ability for people to connect across distances enables groups based around

DOI: 10.4324/9781003391784-2

particular interests to exist, which has opened up a multitude of newly possible communities.

There are many possible ways to describe community.

> A group of people, often living in a defined geographical area, who may share a common culture, values and norms, and are arranged in a social structure according to relationships which the community has developed over a period of time.

is the WHO definition.[2] Communities cross multiple dimensions, whether based on shared values, interests or geography. Members share common needs, beliefs and social norms. Groups are rarely homogenous and almost never mutually exclusive. People belong to many communities at one time, some of which are based around place, at differing scales. Varying degrees of magnification mean localities are nested within a 'hierarchy of place', so that being from a certain part of town leaves at least four possible levels of location: area, town, county and country. We shift between these place identifications depending on context, our social selves varying according to which of these identities is salient at the time. We belong to and influence distinct but overlapping communities, which in turn influence who we are.

## Support

The need for and provision of support is at the heart of our interactions with others, support meaning different things at different times (Table 1.1). Support is a widely used term describing many different types of help, whether offering information, advice, perspective or practical forms of support such as a lift or a loan. Emotional support is a vital part of this, and companionship, someone to confide in, is integral to our wellbeing. Touch brings the physiological benefits of lowered blood pressure and heart rate, causing us to react more positively to others.[3] All of these make up the substance of our interactions, but the common component is the time spent helping each other.

*Table 1.1* Types of support[a]

| | |
| --- | --- |
| Appraisal support | Help with decision-making by providing external perspectives |
| Instrumental support | Practical support, helping with tangible needs |
| Informational support | Advice and information |
| Emotional support | Love and care |

Note:
a Berkman, Lisa F, Glass, Thomas. Social integration, social networks, social support, and health. In: Berkman, Lisa F, Kawachi, Ichiro, eds. *Social Epidemiology*. Oxford Univ. Press; 2000:137–173.

Our social responsibility to each other underpins our sense of belonging. The responsibility for the needs of others as well as our own creates a tension between the individual and the collective, which runs through attempts at defining community as well as much of our political discourse. The *moi humain*, the human 'me' or natural self, shifts towards the *moi commun*, the civic self, individual becoming citizen (Jean-Jacques Rousseau).[4] 'Community is the extent to which one is willing to give up part of the self in order to gain a larger benefit'.[5]

Relationships within communities form archetypes of both traditional associations with emotional attachments and more goal-oriented but less personal interactions. These loosely represent community and society respectively (*gemeinschaft* and *gesellschaft*, Ferdinant Tönnies). These are the links that hold our shared stories together, emotional connections on which our sense of community is built. These interactions reinforce shared values, which in turn translate into social and cultural norms which moderate our behaviour. As we interact with each other, our awareness of our part in the wider social milieu is heightened, increasing our social cohesiveness and forming our shared narrative.

## Groups

Our sense of togetherness and cohesion comes from our awareness of a group identity, an 'us'. All groups define themselves by their boundaries, exclusive definitions we create based around what we are not. While geographies are easily recognisable to all, other commonalities may be less obvious, especially to those outside a group. In areas of high population density, geographic boundaries become less meaningful, so we use other ways to find and establish our tribe, such as shared interests, religion or culture.

'Spirit', the spark of friendship, is an essential element to create and maintain a group.[6] Symbols help to identify members, whether icons and flags or conventions such as dress and language. Similarity, like attracting like (homophily), is a strong factor promoting group formation, but restricted diversity hinders the evolution of groups, which only grow by members challenging norms. Recognising and celebrating differences creates more resilient societies better able to respond to stresses.[7]

Cohesiveness and sense of belonging arise from pressure to conform to a group, individuality traded for the benefits of group membership. This brings security, whether physical, economic or emotional, rewarding personal investment. Membership of multiple groups increases resources, leading to better wellbeing and adaptability.[8] A cohesive community has strong shared values, creating symbiotic benefits reinforcing the group.

Discussing the criteria for group inclusion helps to create and maintain identity and cohesion within the group. There will always be tension at the boundary. Exclusionary approaches may be damaging to those outside the group, sometimes deliberately. Whether by keeping poverty and social justice out of communities or casting out those who deviate from shared norms, limiting inclusion reinforces the group. Some people deliberately exclude themselves to draw attention to an injustice, but a change of direction comes only when a cause is taken up by the more influential members of a group. More representative leadership comes from a fairer distribution of power within the group, through collaboration rather than competition. Good leadership brings out the best in others.

Feeling influential is a strong reinforcing factor for sense of belonging. Group membership brings collective influence, especially to young or marginalised people to whom it would not be individually available. Influence runs both ways, encouraging conformity in members, who in turn determine the direction of the group. Trust is necessary for influence, requiring a sense of order, an understanding of social norms, and a recognition of the authority invested in leaders. Shared principles are sometimes formalised, as with laws and constitutions, but are more often unwritten and outside of our awareness. The way we behave in respect to each other influences our every conversation and interaction, social norms and values constantly remodelled by challenge and reinforcement.

*Table 1.2* Concepts of community

| | |
|---|---|
| Sense of community | Being part of a supportive structure, 'a feeling that members have of belonging, a feeling that members matter to one another and to the group, and a shared faith that members' needs will be met through their commitment to be together'.[a] |
| Sense of coherence | This derives from confidence in resources and structures, the predictability and manageability of our shared circumstances, and a sense of meaning in our shared lives. |
| Social cohesion | The sense of belongingness coming from shared values, which allows community members to cooperate despite differences. |
| Social identity | How we define ourselves in relation to others.[b] |
| Place identification | How residents define a location, especially with regard to the distinctive attributes of a place. |
| Place-related social identity | Formed from the interactions between our physical environment and our social identity, which can be anything from nationalism to pride in one's street.[c] |
| Community capacity / competence | The ability of a community to manage and solve problems of collective life.[b] |

Notes:
a Iyer A, Jetten J, Tsivrikos D, Postmes T, Haslam SA. The more (and the more compatible) the merrier: Multiple group memberships and identity compatibility as predictors of adjustment after life transitions. *Br J Soc Psychol.* 2009;48(4):707–733. doi:10.1348/014466608X397628.
b Tajfel, Henri, Turner, John. The social identity theory of intergroup behaviour. In: Austin WG, Worchel S, eds. *Psychology of Intergroup Relations.* 2nd ed. The Nelson-Hall series in psychology. Nelson-Hall Publishers; 1986.
c McMillan DW, Chavis DM. Sense of community: a definition and theory. *J Community Psychol.* 1986;14(1):6–23.

Community becomes manifest when members act together. Our interpersonal relationships shape our experience of community around us. These ties can be diverse, complex, superficial or deep, but the interconnections join us together, creating a whole that is greater than the sum of the parts. Shared experiences, especially of significant moments, become part of a joint history, which itself reinforces community bonds. A common narrative can be found within the concept of folk spirit, *volksgeist*, the spirit of the people. This invokes national character through cultural contexts such as art and music to create a sense of unity. Collective heritage becomes instantiated in the form of art, and this creativity reinforces the sense of spirit that keeps the community alive.

Our social identities are created by our interactions with others, a continual process adapting the multiple facets of who we are in response to those around us. We have many social identities, which become salient depending on the context. We may identify as a spouse, parent, sibling, child, colleague, friend or stranger, and respond differently depending on which identity is being appealed to. Our social identity, the story other people would tell about us, is reflected by our membership in groups, onto whose norms our own are projected.

Along with membership and social interactions, place is an important component of sense of community. Expectations of behaviour in a physical environment make up our ideas of what a place is (Figure 1.1).[9] A shared sense of place exists in our mental maps, which merge function, history and meaning. Explanations for the way a locality has developed form part of our sense of place, holding collective social meaning. A common narrative, maintained and transformed over generations of neighbourhood discussion, chronicles the essence of a location. Both our history and our present are found within our collective story, told by the community.

Collective action needs social cohesion, place-related social identity and shared needs. Cohesion and social identity are mutually reinforcing. Cohesiveness comes from identifying with a group, increasing cooperative

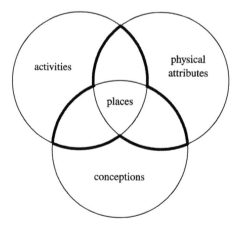

*Figure 1.1* Visual metaphor for the nature of place.

Source: Canter D. *The Psychology of Place*. Architectural Press, 1977.

*Table 1.3* Types of intangible capital

| | |
|---|---|
| Social capital | The extent or value of connections between individuals, a resource that is both societal (Robert Putnam) and individual (Pierre Bourdieu) |
| Community capital | Community assets including relationships |
| Human capital | The expertise of workers |
| Institutional capital | Benefits accrued from strong governance and the laws underpinning an efficient economy |
| Cultural capital | The knowledge, beliefs and attitudes underlying our social structures |
| Linking capital | Connections between individuals and formal institutions |

behaviour and group identification. Self-identifying with the group comes from seeing connections within the group, but also from rejecting that which one is not. This creation of 'otherness' is vulnerable to external pressures, when division is created by highlighting differences rather than common factors.

*Social capital* describes the value of connections among individuals, recognising that the people around us form an essential asset. The various institutions and practices that support our society are held together by the glue of social capital. The use of a term from economics reflects how the value of these connections has been recognised and quantified. Social capital forms part of the intangible assets that make up the wealth of a nation, along with naturally occurring resources and the flow of income derived from those resources. Intangible capital makes up between 60 and 80 per cent of total wealth,[10] more in higher-income countries. Social capital is perpetually renewable and not limited by scarcity, but it atrophies if neglected, needing the maintenance of continued interactions.

## Bridges and bonds

Personal relationships, social networks, civic engagement, cooperative norms and trust all make up social capital. These connections lie at the heart of social networks, the ties of relationships between individuals, which can be horizontal or vertical. Vertical ties, seen in workplaces and gangs, cross the contours of power, offering opportunities and influence within less democratic and more hierarchical structures. Family, neighbourhood and voluntary organisation connections are more horizontal, and are considered *bonding* among people with similar characteristics, or *bridging* when straddling differences, for example across age or ethnicity.[11] Bonding relationships help us get by, bridging ones help us get ahead.

Bonds can be further characterised into strong or weak, with strong bonds such as those within families and between friends maintained frequently. Weak bonds are non-intimate and less frequently refreshed but are no less important. Ideas diffuse further through weak ties, which have more reach ('the strength of weak ties', Mark Granovetter).[12] Innovators tend to be found at the margins, where there is less social pressure to conform. Ideas spread when picked up by those with more ties and stronger bonds.

Bridging and bonding ties help to explain the dynamic between identity and social cohesion. Identity is reinforced more by close, stronger bonds, while social cohesion arises from weaker, bridging ties. Multiplexed connections are those that are duplicated, for example, connections occurring both in and outside of work. In dense or close-knit networks, an individual's friends tend to know each other. Poorer people tend to have proportionately more bonding and fewer bridging relationships. The breadth of bridging ties is strongly associated with educational achievement. Who you know remains an important factor in progression of career or other goals.

A natural experiment occurred in Italy in the 1970s following devolution to regional government, demonstrating the strong link between social capital and economic performance.[13] The economic successes of the more northerly regions were built on strong horizontal ties, where mutual support had been culturally embedded. In the south, patron-client relationships were dominant, and inefficiency and corruption were common within government. The strongest predictor of good governance was the presence of horizontal community groups such as choral societies, soccer clubs and cooperatives. It was not that economic successes had led to increased leisure time, but instead that the presence of these groups exemplified trust and community engagement. The social capital within communities led to prosperity and better governance.

Social capital is not an inherent good, often following existing power structures and keeping the marginalised at the edges. Social networks can be exclusionary, limiting social mobility and restricting resources to a chosen few. This happens when bonding occurs without bridging, leading to isolated cliques. The lack of diversity among political leaders reflects the power of closed networks such as the 'old school tie'. It is not a coincidence that more than a third of UK Prime Ministers in the last two centuries attended the same school. Cultural capital which reinforces privilege and social class by exclusion allows nepotism and corruption to prosper unchallenged.[14]

A sense of being part of a wider whole seems to protect us in times of adversity. Acting in solidarity with the interests of the wider community usually also serves our individual interests.[15] Increased social cohesion reduces suicide rates when a group is exposed to external threats (Émile Durkheim).[16] Pro-social behaviour quickly dominates when a threat is perceived, for instance in response to disasters.[17] Social norms are not only preserved but accentuated, with the less able given protection and disapproval of those who breach these norms. Crowds may already have a common sense of identity such as at football matches, or have no prior connection, but swiftly develop a shared social identity when threatened. This shift from 'me' to 'we' gives collective resilience in situations where acting together improves the chances of self-preservation.

The expression of our collective identity helps to create the 'glue' of social capital. For the moral philosophers of the eighteenth century, *sympathy* was the basis of social harmony. The term 'sympathy' was first used by Galen in the second century to describe the coordination of bodily organs, leading to the names for the sympathetic and parasympathetic drive of the autonomic nervous system, but the meaning developed to include associations or mutual relationships. The economist Adam Smith thought sympathy arose from putting oneself in another's situation, his idea of sympathy deriving from the recognition of our emotions by another. Smith saw the value of a benevolent action as being in the favours it gained from others, but accepted that for some, these social bonds represent altruistic, unselfish acts without expectation of reciprocity.

The natural social order Smith believed in was one where the peace and order of society 'is of more importance than even the relief of the miserable',[18] shaping the future basis of mainstream economics. However, Smith's theories failed to attribute value to unacknowledged work, such as that done by his mother feeding and looking after him.[19] Unpaid core work such as this remains invisible within economic models. Even now, cutting funding for care takes it off the balance sheet and pushes it back into the home, with the burden still picked up predominantly by women, reinforcing gender inequality.

Trust, a component of social capital, makes credit possible, the word coming from the Italian *credo*, to believe. Smith recognised trust as a prerequisite for trade but saw it as coming from the necessity of self-interest, happy to sit back and let the 'invisible hand' of the market distribute resources appropriately. This depersonalised economic view paved the way for game theory, which reduces human interaction to a series of transactions based only on self-interest (John Nash). Game theory suggests there is no need for trust in interactions, and that people will naturally revert to whatever meets their own needs without consideration of others. This has become enshrined in neoliberal thought, celebrating the triumph of individualism over facing challenges collectively.

In fact, people commonly consider the needs of others. Altruistic acts are frequent even when there is no possibility of gain in the future. Empathy is visible in babies, who show emotional arousal in response to the expressions of others. We learn to be helpful through experience and modelling by others, internalising social norms and achieving personal satisfaction through helping. Helping others in distress reduces our own empathetic arousal, but the urge to help also comes from an altruistic motivation, one without anticipation of external reward. The wish to help others who have been treated unfairly is so strong that a cognitive dissonance arises when unable to help. Rather than confront our own lack of power, we instead find reasons to blame victims ('just-world hypothesis').[20]

The evolutionary gain from pro-social behaviours which benefit the wider group explains why these are hard-wired into many species. That individualism has become the default for Western societies has left behind more collaborative approaches, but cooperative behaviours have long been necessary for our survival. Societies have always relied on the benefits of communal living to thrive. Hunter-gathering and farming societies rely on shared approaches for the benefits of scale needed to survive in marginal environments. Social mores and taboos reinforce the expectation of cooperation.

## Individualism

How and when do we start thinking of ourselves as individuals? The coming into being of a sense of self starts as a separation from the universal. Object relations, a branch of psychology which looks at very early infant relationships, suggests that existential distress comes from this estrangement. Realising one's nature as an individual is a loss from wider existence (Melanie Klein), echoing the fall from grace, man's exile from the Garden of Eden.[21] This is a crucial time in our early lives, and the effects of whether our early needs are met ripple on throughout our lives. A parent who is 'good-enough' supports their child to discover that they exist separately, helping them to integrate a sense of self, and ultimately develop the capacity to be alone (Donald Winnicott).[22] Strong boundaries around sense of self are crucial for us to develop healthy relationships, but the rise of the individual in our society has come at the cost of our communal selves.

The tension between individual and collective need is illustrated well by the 'tragedy of the commons'.[23] This was originally a thought experiment to describe the harm done from overgrazing shared land.[24] While it may be in an individual's interest to graze more animals on shared land to maximise individual returns, excessive stock damages the land and undermines the common interest. The same principles apply wherever costs can be externalised, bringing individual gain even though everyone pays more overall. This has been used as an argument for privatising shared assets, despite numerous examples of successfully self-regulating commons.

Elinor Ostrom won the Nobel Prize for economics by showing that communication builds trust, leading to the sustainable management of local environments and resources. Community ownership models are not only self-sustaining but more efficient than monopolies. She demonstrated the resilience of diverse, interlocking institutions in communities where autonomy and trust can flourish.[25] These are built on *subsidiarity*, the principle by which decisions should be taken at the most local level possible, which makes for effective local governance.

The idea of the primacy of the individual coincided with the rise of a trading class. Itinerant traders made profit by moving goods which could be sold at higher cost. Along with moneylenders, these outsiders were less trusted by communities, although being outside of traditional community structures made cooperation less important.[26] Those without a strong community will prefer to prioritise individual values over collective ones.

Sigmund Freud's ideas on the development of the ego were used to promote the individual as the primary unit of society. Freud's nephew, Edward Bernays, used his uncle's work to identify the ways in which we are manipulable, allowing others influence over our behaviour. The manufacturing industry, hugely scaled up for wartime effort, was left at risk of overproduction when war ended, so a need was created for consumption to fill, presenting purchasing as a patriotic duty. Bernays created the modern PR industry to promote individualism as a way to market products to consumers. Psychology became a tool of commerce, eroding our sense of self to influence our behaviour.

## Media

Media, both traditional and social, contribute much of our sense of who we are. Television is associated with far less social capital than newspaper reading (Robert Putnam).[27] The spread of television saw a steady decline in civic engagement, which had peaked in the 1920s. Television channels serve wide areas, making content less likely to be locally relevant, so effects on sense of cohesion are less place-based. Content matters; using media to access information increases social capital, while entertainment boosts networking capital but not civic engagement.[28] Sitcoms reinforce trust by modelling interpersonal relationships, but fictional portrayals of a mean world increase social mistrust.

The rise of social media has made it easy to micropublish online, bringing the unprecedented ability to communicate with anyone interested, opening up potential connections across the globe. Updates can be published instantly, and this ease of communication increases connectedness, which in turn builds interpersonal trust. Users are now the main content creators, inverting previous top-down media and democratising the control of information. Blog readers who are active online tend also to be active participants offline.[29] The ability to coordinate protests and online petitions has aided a change from 'dutiful citizen' to 'actualising citizen',[30] whose personal values are expressed within a loose network of social activism.

Internet use in general is associated with greater civic engagement.[31] Overall frequency of social networking sites (SNS) use is not related to civic participation,[32] but instead, as with traditional media, increased participation arises from the way in which SNS are used. Using SNS to find information significantly predicts both online and offline civic engagement. Material that has been filtered and curated by peers is more trusted, the ease of interactivity helping to generate reflective dialogue.

Social media and internet use can still be exclusionary. The stigma of being a newcomer and the jargon used can be off-putting to new users. Wider interactions increase the risk of exposure to unpleasant exchanges, which can be distressing even for those with strong support networks. Sites which hide content behind access controls limit the flow of information and hinder wider connections. SNS companies have a vested interest in keeping users within their sites, appropriating and enclosing the commons their users create.

The ease of generating these new non-geographic ties leads to far wider and potentially more diverse networks, reaching across different platform architectures which generate varying patterns of engagement.[33] For instance, Twitter's ability to follow and copy in any other user encourages bridging ties, while other sites are orientated more towards bonding with those already familiar to us. This is changing as sites develop their audiences. Facebook started as a way to keep in touch with people already known to us but is increasingly used for bridging.[34]

Connected users tend to be similar, often considered to be in the same 'bubble'. Users with this higher homophily have more bonding connections, while connections between those with more heterogeneous peer groups are

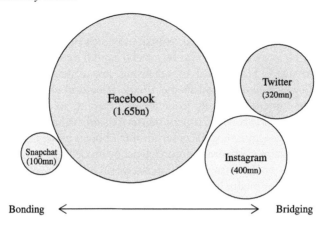

*Figure 1.2* Bonding and bridging on social networking sites (size shows number of regular users).

Source: Phua J, Jin SV, Kim J (Jay). Uses and gratifications of social networking sites for bridging and bonding social capital: a comparison of Facebook, Twitter, Instagram, and Snapchat. *Comput Hum Behav*. 2017;72:115–122. doi:10.1016/j.chb.2017.02.041.

more bridging.[35] These different types of ties affect the way we interact on social networking sites, and the way these sites interact with us.

## Social capital and health

These bonds and bridges, whether online, in our homes and workplaces or elsewhere, all have an influence on our health. Social capital is not so much created by individuals as existing in the spaces between us. Some of the benefits realised are manifestly public, such as trust and shared values, but social capital also improves the health of individuals and communities.

Many studies have shown a link between better health outcomes and enhanced social capital. Individual level social capital is strongly associated with better self-reported health,[36] partly as a result of improved access to health information via more plentiful interactions. Connected groups are better able to advocate for healthcare and have increased access to informal support and care.

Inequality damages the health of the population by eroding social cohesion.[37] Social capital has less influence on health in more equal societies. Individual social capital is the main determinant of health, but only in the presence of community social capital.[38] In this sense, it is community social capital such as trust that catalyses the benefits to individuals.

Trust is an important component of social capital, with better health in countries where there is more trust between people.[39] Increases in trust, reciprocity and civic participation are all strongly associated with lower mortality.[40] Behaviours spread via social networks, affecting people who may not be connected directly. This makes network-based interventions an effective way to modulate harmful behaviours. Quitting smoking, for example, diffuses across networks, individual behaviours influenced by intermediaries which leave smokers marginalised.[41]

Participation needs trust, which is built on social connections. The strongest predictor of civic engagement is higher educational status, followed by increasing age.[42] Participation, whether volunteering and voting, reduces the chance of cardiovascular disease.[43] Community development benefits all members of a community, but the greatest health benefits go to individuals who are actively participating.[44]

## Measuring social capital

Quantifying social capital depends very much on what aspects are being examined. Social networks, for instance, can be described in terms of their range, density, boundedness, homogeneity, frequency of contact, multiplexity, duration and reciprocity.[45] A local estimate of social capital can be derived from publicly available data on associated factors.[46]

*Table 1.4* Measures of social capital

| | |
|---|---|
| Social capital | ONS survey in the UK measures personal relationships, social network support, civic engagement and trust and cooperative norms[a] |
| | Co-op community wellbeing index[b] |
| | Social Capital Questionnaire[c] |
| Values | World Values Survey surveying values, beliefs and norms across 120 countries worldwide[d] |
| Sense of community | SCI-1, Sense of Community Index, neighbourhood survey giving a 12-point score of agreement with statements about neighbourhood, mapping onto membership, influence, needs and shared emotional connection[e] |
| Civic | Freedom House scores reflect political rights and civil liberties in countries across the world over five decades[f] |
| | Gastil index of political and civil rights for countries |
| Economic | The total value of voluntary activity in the UK is estimated at £24 bn, representing 1.5 per cent of GDP[g] |

a  Office for National Statistics. *Social Capital in the UK: April 2020 to March 2021*. ONS; 2022. https://www.ons.gov.uk/peoplepopulationandcommunity/wellbeing/bulletins/socialcapitalintheuk/april2020tomarch2021

b  Berkman, Lisa F, Glass, Thomas. Social integration, social networks, social support, and health. In: Berkman, Lisa F, Kawachi, Ichiro, eds. *Social Epidemiology*. Oxford Univ. Press; 2000:137–173.

c  Onyx J, Bullen P. Measuring social capital in five communities. *J Appl Behav Sci*. 2000;36(1):23–42. doi:10.1177/0021886300361002.

d  World Values Survey. https://www.worldvaluessurvey.org/wvs.jsp

e  Perkins DD, Florin P, Rich RC, Wandersman A, Chavis DM. Participation and the social and physical environment of residential blocks: crime and community context. *Am J Community Psychol*. 1990;18(1):83–115. doi:10.1007/BF00922690.

f  Freedom in the World. Freedom House. https://freedomhouse.org/report/freedom-world

g  Office for National Statistics. *Household Satellite Accounts - Valuing Voluntary Activity in the Uk*. ONS;2013. http://www.ons.gov.uk/ons/rel/wellbeing/household-satellite-accounts/valuing-voluntary-activity-in-the-uk/art--valuing-voluntary-activity-in-the-uk.html

Social capital is health-enabling, and outcomes are worse when it is lacking. Aspects of our shared lives such as loneliness and discrimination interact with our physiology, amplifying risk factors which affect our health. Being with others increases our wellbeing, our resources and improves our health. Building social capital is health-creating. To understand how, we need to explore what health is and what makes us healthy.

## Notes

Links and additional resources for this chapter can be found at www.communityhealth. uk/1-community-health

1 WHO Centre for Health Development. *A Glossary of Terms for Community Health Care and Services for Older Persons.* Vol 5. World Health Organization; 2004. https://apps.who.int/iris/handle/10665/68896

2 Ibid.

3 Gallace A, Spence C. The science of interpersonal touch: an overview. *Neurosci Biobehav Rev.* 2010;34(2):246–259. doi:10.1016/j.neubiorev.2008.10.004.

4 Shklar, Judith N. *Men and Citizens: A Study of Rousseau's Social Theory.* Cambridge University Press; 1969.

5 Patrick, Donald, Wickizer, Thomas. Community and Health. In: Amick B, Levine, Sol, Tarlov, Alvin, Chapman Walsh, Diana, eds. *Society and Health.* Oxford University Press; 1995:46–92.

6 McMillan DW. Sense of community. *J Community Psychol.* 1996;24(4):315–325.

7 Eachus P. Community resilience: is it greater than the sum of the parts of individual resilience? *Procedia Econ Finance.* 2014;18:345–351. doi:10.1016/S2212-5671(14)00949-6.

8 Iyer A, Jetten J, Tsivrikos D, Postmes T, Haslam SA. The more (and the more compatible) the merrier: Multiple group memberships and identity compatibility as predictors of adjustment after life transitions. *Br J Soc Psychol.* 2009;48(4):707–733. doi:10.1348/014466608X397628.

9 Canter D. *The Psychology of Place.* Architectural Press; 1977.

10 World Bank. *The Changing Wealth of Nations: Measuring Sustainable Development in the New Millennium.*; 2011. https://openknowledge.worldbank.org/handle/10986/2252

11 Ferlander S. The importance of different forms of social capital for health. *Acta Sociol.* 2007;50(2):115–128. doi:10.1177/0001699307077654.

12 Granovetter MS. The strength of weak ties. *Am J Sociol.* 1973;78(6):1360–1380. doi:10.1086/225469.

13 Putnam RD. What makes democracy work? *Natl Civ Rev.* 1993;82(2):101–107. doi:10.1002/ncr.4100820204.

14 Bourdieu, Pierre. The forms of capital. In: *Richardson, J, Handbook of Theory and Research for the Sociology of Education.* Greenwood; 1986:241–258.

15 Tudor Hart J. *The Political Economy of Health Care: A Clinical Perspective.* The Policy Press; 2006.

16 Durkheim, Émile. *Suicide: A Study in Sociology.* Routledge; 1897.

17 Drury, John. Collective resilience in mass emergencies and disasters: a social identity model. In: *The Social Cure: Identity, Health and Well-Being.* Psychology Press; 2012:195–215.

18 Smith, Adam. *The Theory of Moral Sentiments.* Andrew Millar; 1759.

19 Raworth, Kate. *Doughnut Economics: Seven Ways to Think Like a 21st-Century Economist.* Random House; 2017.

20 Lerner MJ. *The Belief in a Just World: A Fundamental Delusion.*; 1980.

21  Hunt J. Psychological perspectives on the garden of Eden and the fall in light of the work of Melanie Klein and Eric Fromm. *Pastor Psychol.* 2018;67(1):33–41. doi:10.1007/s11089-017-0790-0.

22  Winnicott DW. The capacity to be alone. *Int J Psychoanal.* 1958;39(5):416–420. doi:10.1093/med:psych/9780190271374.003.0060.

23  Ostrom E. Coping with tragedies of the commons. *Annu Rev Polit Sci.* 1999;2(1):493–535. doi:10.1146/annurev.polisci.2.1.493.

24  Hardin G. The tragedy of the commons: the population problem has no technical solution; it requires a fundamental extension in morality. *Science.* 1968;162(3859):1243–1248. doi:10.1126/science.162.3859.1243.

25  Kaye, Simon. *Thing Big, Act Small: Elinor Ostrom's Radical Vision for Community Power.* New Local; 2020. https://www.newlocal.org.uk/publications/ostrom/

26  Lerner M. *Surplus Powerlessness: The Psychodynamics of Everyday Life – and the Psychology of Individual and Social Transformation.* Institute for Labor & Mental Health; 1986.

27  Putnam RD. Tuning in, tuning out: the strange disappearance of social capital in America. *PS Polit Sci Polit.* 1995;28(4):664. doi:10.2307/420517.

28  Geber S, Scherer H, Hefner D. Social capital in media societies: The impact of media use and media structures on social capital. *Int Commun Gaz.* 2016;78(6):493–513. doi:10.1177/1748048516640211.

29  Gil de Zúñiga H, Veenstra A, Vraga E, Shah D. Digital democracy: reimagining pathways to political participation. *J Inf Technol Polit.* 2010;7(1):36–51. doi:10.1080/19331680903316742.

30  Bennett, W. Lance. Changing citizenship in the digital age. In: Bennett WL, ed. *Civic Life Online: Learning How Digital Media Can Engage Youth.* The John D. and Catherine T. Macarthur Foundation series on digital media and learning. MIT Press; 2008. doi:10.7551/mitpress/7893.003.0002.

31  Wellman B, Haase AQ, Witte J, Hampton K. Does the internet increase, decrease, or supplement social capital? Social networks, participation, and community commitment. *Am Behav Sci.* 2001;45(3):436–455. doi:10.1177/00027640121957286.

32  Gil de Zúñiga H, Jung N, Valenzuela S. Social media use for news and individuals' social capital, civic engagement and political participation. *J Comput-Mediat Commun.* 2012;17(3):319–336. doi:10.1111/j.1083-6101.2012.01574.x.

33  Phua J, Jin SV, Kim J (Jay). Uses and gratifications of social networking sites for bridging and bonding social capital: a comparison of Facebook, Twitter, Instagram, and Snapchat. *Comput Hum Behav.* 2017;72:115–122. doi:10.1016/j.chb.2017.02.041.

34  Alhabash S, Ma M. A tale of four platforms: motivations and uses of Facebook, Twitter, Instagram, and Snapchat among college students? *Soc Media Soc.* 2017;3(1):205630511769154. doi:10.1177/2056305117691544.

35  See note 33.

36  Kim, Daniel, Subramanian, S., Kawachi, Ichiro. Social capital and physical health. In: Kawachi I, Subramanian S, Kim D, eds. *Social Capital and Health.* Springer New York; 2010:139–190.

37  Kawachi, Ichiro, Subramanian, S., Kim, Daniel. Social capital and health. In: Kawachi I, Subramanian S, Kim D, eds. *Social Capital and Health.* Springer New York; 2010:1–26.

38  Rocco, Lorenzo, Suhrcke, Marc. *Is Social Capital Good for Health? A European Perspective.* World Health Organisation Regional Office for Europe; 2012. https://apps.who.int/iris/bitstream/handle/10665/352821/9789289002738-eng.pdf

39  Ibid.

40  Lochner KA, Kawachi I, Brennan RT, Buka SL. Social capital and neighborhood mortality rates in Chicago. *Soc Sci Med.* 2003;56(8):1797–1805. doi:10.1016/S0277-9536(02)00177-6.

41  Christakis NA, Fowler JH. The collective dynamics of smoking in a large social network. *N Engl J Med*. 2008;358(21):2249–2258. doi:10.1056/NEJMsa0706154.
42  See note 27.
43  See note 36.
44  See note 40.
45  Berkman, Lisa F, Glass, Thomas. Social integration, social networks, social support, and health. In: Berkman, Lisa F, Kawachi, Ichiro, eds. *Social Epidemiology*. Oxford Univ. Press; 2000:137–173.
46  Hill-Dixon, Amanda, Solley, Suzanne, Bynon, Radhika. *Being Well Together: The Creation of the Co-Op Community Wellbeing Index*. The Young Foundation; 2020. https://communitywellbeing.coop.co.uk/community-wellbeing-index-reports/

# 2 Health and its determinants

The term *health* can mean many things. Health is defined by the WHO as a 'state of complete physical, mental and social wellbeing'.[1] Few of us would meet this definition, which casts the majority of us as unhealthy, even if we do not notice any limitations. We learn to tolerate our restrictions, on the whole. We find out the hard way what we can do, and what our bodies will not let us get away with. After a while, goalposts shift, and we stop doing the things that cause us problems. Most of us accept the consequences of physical changes due to ageing as a trade-off for living longer. This is not a state of health, according to the WHO, yet there are no symptoms. Can someone with disease but without symptoms be healthy? Striving constantly for an ideal leads to medicalisation and interventions of minimal benefit. A definition based on a state of perfection harms those with illness or disability, both assuming and devaluing their experience of their bodies.

The other way to define health is by that which it is not. The healthy body is transparent (Jean-Paul Sartre), becoming visible when we are unwell.[2] The boundary between health and illness shifts constantly depending on the context. Health is experienced by individuals, or more accurately, health is not experienced by individuals; it is poor health that takes our attention, as the absence of illness goes unnoticed. Symptoms are what are experienced, bodily sensations that we become aware of, usually arising from physiological changes. Our bodies are always feeding back to us, whether we choose to focus on that feeling or not. Coenaesthesia, the awareness of our bodies, is how being alive feels. You are feeling it now. Being healthy is the ability to forget about one's body.[3]

## Illness and disease

The context in which our symptoms are experienced shapes our reactions, influenced as they are by our internalised concepts, cultural norms and the responses of the people around us. This 'social architecture of illness'[4] provides a context for our symptoms, framing them in terms of illness and disease. These are overlapping concepts, representing ways of constructing reality. Illness is the subjective experience of poor health, while disease describes the objective findings. Put most simply, patients go to the doctor

DOI: 10.4324/9781003391784-3

*Table 2.1* Antonovsky's conceptual model of health[a]

| Non-patient | Healthy | |
|---|---|---|
| | Sick | Not yet diagnosed |
| | | Specific, diagnosable illness |
| Patient | Disease | Symptomatic |
| | | Diagnosed |
| | No disease | Malingering |

Note:
a Antonovsky, Aaron. *Health, Stress and Coping.* Jossey-Bass; 1979.

with illness and leave with disease.[5] It is possible to have a disease without symptoms, and symptoms without disease. Some conditions are asymptomatic, especially in early stages. Bodily sensations presented as potential symptoms are often unrelated to any underlying disease process.

Antovosky's schema (Table 2.1) demonstrates the flaws in thinking about health as the presence or absence of disease. A person can be sick or healthy, patient or not, but forcing a label of malingering onto those in a patient role without disease lacks understanding of the social context of symptoms, and the role of healthcare in turning people into patients.

Noticing our bodies is the reason that people seek healthcare. We mostly assume our bodies will continue to work as they always have, so we notice only when something seems wrong. Our bodies demand our attention, and at some point a decision to seek help is made, usually when those symptoms impact on the individual or those around them. This is where the boundaries of health lie. The act of seeking help begins a new narrative, which needs resolution for healing to occur. Asking for external help brings those symptoms into a reality shared with others.

These sensations, initially unexplained, can be put together in various ways, one of which becomes the dominant narrative of the illness. The art of clinical practice is in exploring these alternative narratives, uncovering stories which allow healing.

Illness becomes disease when it is named. This explains, delimits and frames symptoms into a context which is culturally coherent, but de-emphasises the experience of the patient.[6] The nature of the relationship with symptoms changes once these are attributed to disease. Becoming a patient brings a change in social identity, subjecting us to cultural expectations of how we should be as we enter the sanctum of healthcare.

A consultation with a practitioner involves coming to a shared understanding that reconciles the patient's illness state with the practitioner's concepts of disease. Lay and professional beliefs must meet in the common ground between ethnomedical and biomedical concepts for this dialogue to take place. Folk beliefs around health usually explain ill health as being due to one of four main processes: *invasion,* such as by germs or cancer; *degeneration,* being run down; *mechanical* systems liable to blockages; and *balance* or the lack of it, such as of vitamins or sleep.[7] Most consultations at some level reflect concern about one of these, although this is a two-way process, with clinicians also invoking these explanations to share understanding. Different medical systems share modalities of treatments, usually based on activity, medicines, behaviours or physical interventions. Treatments based on activity can vary from prescribed exercise to bed rest. Medicines are applied or ingested, while behaviours such as prayers and talking therapies or interventions such as surgery can be prescribed.

The consultation itself has healing power. The act of telling someone else about symptoms involves acknowledging these to ourselves as being of note. Active listening validates concerns, and reassurance by a clinician often lets symptoms pass back out of notice. The power of the consultation is well recognised in clinical practice, known as 'doctor as drug' (Michael Balint).[8] As with any medicine, there are potential side effects, including dependency.

Defining illness means quantifying it. Criteria are chosen on which to define a diagnosis, which also provides a way to measure the impact. The measures used inevitably determine the results. Laboratory tests are helpful in measuring disease activity, providing proxy markers that quantify physiological changes, but not how these translate into symptoms. Test results can be treated without addressing the symptoms the patient presented with. Patient questionnaires can be used to quantify ill health. Judging the success of treatment on parameters that are defined by patients ensures the practitioner's aims align with those of the patient, redefining and relocating health to the patient instead of the system.

The treatment burden of an illness is the measure patients notice most. Treatment burden describes the cost to the patient, in time, money and the side effects of treatment. Having treatment or waiting for it eats into our lives as patients, whether applying ointments or dressings, sitting in waiting rooms or on hospital transport, or waiting for the date for the next appointment.

Health is highly valued, rated the top priority for people aged 35 and over, above education and life satisfaction.[9] Effort expended on avoiding the burden of disease is worthwhile. Individually and societally, we invest significant resources and time on prevention and treatment. Ensuring interventions are appropriate, cost-effective and beneficial is a fundamental tenet of healthcare, though the dominance of expensive, reactive medicine has unbalanced attempts to improve the health of our populations. Rebalancing medicine means looking anew at the causes of poor health, and ensuring resources get to where they are most effective.

## Social determinants of health

The conditions in which we live have a substantial influence on our health. Our environment, upbringing and circumstances such as income, employment and housing all affect our health. There are large discrepancies in the control that people have over their circumstances, which translate into very different outcomes.

The idea that health is a function of society is woven through the history of medicine. Investigating a typhus epidemic in 1848, Rudolf Virchow showed that while crop failures had led to famine, the poor had been most susceptible. He identified that oppression by aristocracy and bureaucracy together with a lack of education had led to this vulnerability, and recognised that it would be impossible to treat disease without treating the inequalities that led to it.

Virchow, considered the father of social medicine, was an ardent anti-racist and reformist, calling politics 'nothing but medicine at a larger scale'.[10] Virchow's breakthrough was to show disease as normal processes altered by abnormal circumstances. Asking 'Do we not always find the diseases of the populace traceable to defects in society?' he introduced the idea that a population itself can be sick. The way in which we live together, and our interactions with others form a crucial part of what constitutes our health. When our society is less healthy, we are less healthy.

The conditions in which people are born, grow, live, work and age influence health through a complex set of interactions. Socioeconomic factors, education, the effects of social and physical environments as well as access to healthcare, justice and equity all determine health outcomes. These *social determinants of health* (SDOH) hugely impact our health at individual, group and community levels (Table 2.2). These could equally be called political determinants, as they are sensitive to policy decisions. Addressing collective risk factors requires interventions at a collective level.

The most important hard health outcomes – illness, mortality and life expectancy, together with health status and healthcare costs – are all influenced by social determinants, in particular the effects of inequality. Quantifying the enormous impact of social determinants makes the importance of addressing these factors clear.

Cardiovascular disease, which kills more than one in ten people in the UK, is a good example of the causes of the causes. Coronary heart disease is due to arterial damage from inflammation, which is aggravated by stress, deprivation, inequality and loneliness, meaning that social factors are strongly linked to outcomes. Some risk factors such as age, sex and family history are not modifiable. Others, such as inactivity, smoking, poor sugar control and high

*Table 2.2* Social determinants of health

| | |
|---|---|
| Socioeconomic | Employment, income, social status |
| Education | Healthy child development, literacy, vocational training/higher education, access to digital technology |
| Health-related | Nutrition, coping skills, access to services |
| Social environment | Support networks, discrimination, safety, equity |
| Physical environment | Housing, transport, safety, greenspace |

*Table 2.3* NHS costs of modifiable risk factors

| Risk factor | Annual NHS cost[a,b,c,d] |
|---|---|
| Poor diet | £6.0 bn |
| Obesity/overweight | £5.0 bn |
| Smoking | £3.3 bn |
| Alcohol | £3.3 bn |
| Poor housing | £1.4 bn |
| Inactivity | £0.9 bn |

Notes:
a  Rayner M. The burden of food related ill health in the UK. *J Epidemiol Community Health.* 2005;59(12):1054–1057. doi:10.1136/jech.2005.036491.
b  Pretty J, Barton J, Pervez Bharucha Z, et al. Improving health and well-being independently of GDP: dividends of greener and prosocial economies. *Int J Environ Health Res.* 2016;26(1):11–36. doi:10.1080/09603123.2015.1007841.
c  Wilkinson RG. Socioeconomic determinants of health: health inequalities: relative or absolute material standards? *BMJ.* 1997;314(7080):591–591. doi:10.1136/bmj.314.7080.591.
d  Fitzpatrick S, Bramley G, Blenkinsopp J, et al. *Destitution in the UK.* Joseph Rowntree Foundation; 2020. https://www.jrf.org.uk/report/destitution-uk-2020

blood pressure are modifiable risk factors that can be addressed through a combination of individual and societal approaches. Diabetes and high blood pressure both double the risk of cardiovascular disease,[11] but the impact of deprivation is greater; people from the most deprived quintile have a mortality rate nearly three times that of those in the least deprived.[12] Cardiovascular mortality in people who are in contact with mental health services is even higher.[13] Addressing these risk factors substantially reduces healthcare costs (Table 2.3).

## Inequality

Deprivation and inequality affect all our lives. In England, those living in the poorest areas die seven years earlier than those in the richest, who enjoy an extra seventeen years of disability-free life. If everyone in England did as well as the best, over 2 million lost years of life would be restored.[14]

Mortality rates are higher in more unequal societies.[15] The UK has very high income inequality, money trickling up instead of down. While COVID-19 saw a doubling of the wealth of the richest ten people, over a million UK households were unable to afford the absolute essentials of food, shelter and sanitation before the pandemic.[16] Levels of child poverty in the UK were described by the UN Rapporteur as 'a disgrace'.[17] The cost of living is soaring, and poverty has increased by a third since 2017, with more than one in five people in the UK now in poverty.[18]

Healthy choices are harder to make for poorer people; people in the lowest income decile would need to spend two-thirds of their disposable income to follow healthy eating guidance.[19] The local environment is worse in deprived areas, with higher crime and air pollution, and more outlets providing unhealthy services and goods such as gambling, fast food, alcohol and tobacco.[20] Inequality is damaging for society, affecting all, not just those at the bottom of the income gradient. It is expensive to maintain an unequal society, costing more in welfare and healthcare as well as lost taxes.

The communities and places in which we live have an enormous impact on our health. The circumstances around us influence our risk of disease, the patterns visible down to neighbourhood-level data. Average life expectancy drops as one travels further out of affluent central London into the poorer surrounding areas. Algorithms based on real time health data can predict risk of disease down to postcode level (Table 2.4).[21]

Poorer people use more healthcare, are less likely to participate in screening or immunisation and have worse health outcomes.[22] Good medical care is less available to populations with greater need, especially when exposed to market forces (the inverse care law).[23] Decades of improvements in life expectancy have stalled, with life expectancy actually falling for those born in the early 1970s.[24]

*Table 2.4* Poverty and inequality in the UK

| | |
|---|---|
| Inequality | The richest 10% of households have 44% of all wealth in the UK, more than five times the combined wealth of the poorer 50%.[a] |
| Poverty | 14.5 million people are in poverty in the UK, including one in three children. Nearly one in two lone parents is in poverty.[b] |
| Cost of inequality | The worsened outcomes due to these inequalities come at a significant financial cost to the economy, losing up to £32 bn in England annually in welfare and lost taxes, another £31 bn in lost productivity, and an NHS cost of at least £5.5 bn.[c]<br>2.6 million years of life would be gained in the UK by reducing health inequalities.[d] |
| Mortality | Child mortality from external causes is fifteen times more in the lowest compared with the highest social class.[e] |

Notes:
a Office for National Statistics. *Wealth in Great Britain Wave 5: 2014 to 2016*. ONS; 2018. https://www.ons.gov.uk/peoplepopulationandcommunity/personalandhouseholdfinances/incomeandwealth/bulletins/wealthingreatbritainwave5/2014to2016
b Barry, Andrea, Brook, Paul, Cebula, Carla, et al. *UK Poverty 2022*. Joseph Rowntree Foundation; 2022. https://www.jrf.org.uk/report/uk-poverty-2022
c Frontier Economics. *Estimating the Costs of Health Inequalities: A Report Prepared for the Marmot Review*. Frontier Economics Ltd; 2010. https://www.instituteofhealthequity.org/file-manager/FSHLrelateddocs/overall-costs-fshl.pdf
d Popay J, Whitehead M, Hunter DJ. Injustice is killing people on a large scale – but what is to be done about it? *J Public Health*. 2010;32(2):148–149. doi:10.1093/pubmed/fdq029
e Edwards P, Roberts I, Green J, Lutchmun S. Deaths from injury in children and employment status in family: analysis of trends in class specific death rates. *BMJ*. 2006;333(7559):119. doi:10.1136/bmj.38875.757488.4F

The fact that health disparities by income persist in the UK, despite a national health service available to all and free at the point of use, shows how limited medicine can be against the effects of discrimination and poverty. These become self-reinforcing circles; poor health impacts criminal justice, employment and our environment, which in turn affects our health.

Racial prejudice is more common in unequal societies and is associated with worse health outcomes for all. This 'structural violence' leads to higher crime rates, more homicides and more conflict experienced by children.[25] It is not just health and crime that are affected by inequality; unequal societies also do worse in economic terms. Higher share of income among the richest is associated with poorer economic growth.[26] Growth is stimulated by policies that redistribute income from the top to middle-income earners.[27]

The interests of the rich diverge from those of the poor as the difference between them increases. Societies which tolerate large income disparities invest less in healthcare and human capital,[28] disproportionately affecting poorer people. The systemic causes that lead to inequality live within biases in the infrastructure which reduce the resources available to people with low incomes. The poorest pay the greatest proportion of disposable income as tax.[29]

While absolute level of income is strongly linked to health outcomes, relative inequality within a society also seems to damage health. Even when needs are met, differences in income still affect health outcomes. Infant mortality rates and life expectancy are more sensitive to relative than absolute income differences.[30] Societies are stratified by social status, even when income is enough to meet health needs. Being lower in the social hierarchy worsens cardiovascular risk factors.[31] Death rates increase when inequality is higher.[32]

Equality improves the health of all. Income equality and the strength of community life are closely correlated.[33] More equal societies are also more cohesive,[34] and increased social capital is strongly health-generating. The principles of 'liberty, equality and fraternity' were hard won, and empowerment, social status and relationships remain crucial to our health.

Measuring inequality shows how social gradient affects health outcomes. Inequality can be quantified by income, pay or wealth. Income includes other sources of money received as well as pay, while wealth counts total assets. In a society with an equal distribution of wealth, a graph of wealth by population share would increase linearly, making a straight line of equality. But wealth is far from evenly distributed, and in reality the money lies bunched up at one end of the population. Known as a *Lorenz curve* (Figure 2.1), the line of wealth lags far below the line of equality. The difference between the line of equality and the actual distribution is measured for countries as the *Gini coefficient* (Table 2.5). This measure of wealth inequality strongly correlates with higher mortality.[35] The Palma ratio and Robin Hood index are alternative measures of the inequality in a country (Figure 2.2a–c).

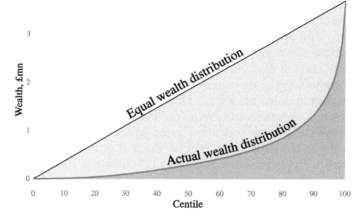

*Figure 2.1* Lorenz curve: Household wealth distribution, Great Britain 2018–2020 Office for National Statistics. Dataset: Household total wealth by percentiles, Great Britain, April 2018 to March 2020. Published online January 7, 2022.

*Table 2.5* Measures of inequality

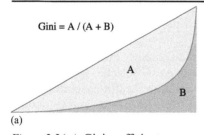

(a)

*Figure 2.2(a)* Gini coefficient.

The Gini coefficient measures the difference between perfect equality and the cumulative share of wealth across a population.

0 is perfect equality, 1 is perfect inequality.

UK Gini is 0.6, implying that 60% of the country's wealth is missing from a fair share (Figure 2.2a).

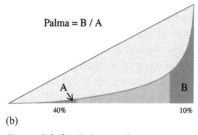

(b)

*Figure 2.2(b)* Palma ratio.

The Palma ratio compares the income share of the top 10% of earners with the lowest 40%,[a] which may reflect inequality more accurately than Gini. A completely equal society would have a Palma ratio of 0.25. The UK Palma ratio is 1.6 (Figure 2.2b).

(*Continued*)

*Table 2.5* (Continued)

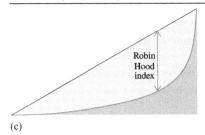

(c)

*Figure 2.2(c)* Robin Hood index.

Robin Hood index is the proportion of income that would have to be shared by households above the mean with those below the mean to distribute income equally. Graphically, the maximum difference between the line of equality and Lorenz curve.
44% of UK wealth would have to be transferred from rich to poor to achieve equality. Each 1% increase in the Robin Hood index is associated with 21 extra deaths per 100,000 people per year (Figure 2.2c).[b]

Index of Multiple Deprivation

Local measure of deprivation combining 37 indicators across 7 domains, covering income, employment, education and skills, health, crime, housing and environment, providing a relative ranking of deprivation.

Notes:
a  Cobham A, Sumner A. Is inequality all about the tails? The Palma measure of income inequality. *Significance*. 2014;11(1):10–13. doi:10.1111/j.1740-9713.2014.00718.x.
b  Kennedy BP, Kawachi I, Prothrow-Stith D. Income distribution and mortality: cross sectional ecological study of the Robin Hood index in the United States. *BMJ*. 1996;312(7037):1004–1007. doi:10.1136/bmj.312.7037.1004.

## How do social determinants affect health?

It is abundantly clear that a poor start in life has significant and lifelong repercussions on health status. Adult health is strongly dependent on conditions in the womb. Poor placental function restricts intrauterine growth, with smoking and conditions such as diabetes worsening placental blood flow. The foetal origins of adult disease (Barker) hypothesis explains the link between low birth weight and vascular disease in adulthood as being due to poor nutrition *in utero*, which increases the risk of diabetes and heart disease later in life.[36] Also known as the 'thrifty phenotype', limited availability of nutrients primes the metabolism of the infant to cope with a resource-poor environment in later life. An individual set to cope with scarcity is less able to deal with excess. Plasticity, the ability to adapt to the environment, becomes less pronounced with age. Wartime rationing and subsequent changes in nutrition as societies become more affluent have had long-lasting effects on the health of a generation.

## Microbiome

Our environment also influences our health through effects on the commensal bacteria that live alongside and within us. We each live with a hundred trillion organisms from five hundred or so different species of bacteria, known as the microbiome, residing on our skin and in our respiratory tracts, intestines and orifices. Up to 2 per cent of our body weight consists of these predominantly beneficial bacteria, helping us to digest food and regulate our immune systems. The mix of these differs for every individual, our microbiome carrying a unique signature which is far more diverse than our DNA. Genetics makes only a small contribution, with significant variation even between identical twins.

The influence of very early exposure to the bacteria we live with seems to be important. The microbiome is acquired in infancy and established by the age of two.[37] The maternal environment influences the foetus by changing the composition of the developing microbiome. It was previously thought that meconium, the first stool of an infant, was sterile, but some colonisation occurs while in the womb from the maternal digestive tract via the amniotic fluid. Further transmission occurs during birth, varying by route of delivery. Weaning choices, and the availability of clean water and adequate sanitation, establish a lasting microbiome, with long-term impacts on health.

Gut bacteria play an important role in health, influencing the absorption of nutrients and production of hormones such as serotonin.[38] Environment, diet and antibiotics all affect the composition of the microbiome. Breastfeeding encourages beneficial bacteria, while dysbiosis, an imbalance of gut bacteria, leads to inflammation and poor nutrient absorption. Chronic inflammation and infection such as that from periodontal (gum) disease worsens dysbiosis. Lower bacterial diversity and higher enzyme activity speed up digestion of food, making calories more easily available. This contributes to the obesogenic environment, leading to differences in weight gain. Use of antibiotics in the first six months of life leads to increased body mass in childhood, even when adjusted for other risk factors such as maternal weight and socioeconomic status.[39] Cancer, allergy and autoimmune diseases such as diabetes have all been linked to an unhealthy microbiome.[40] The balance of our microbiome changes according to food choices, a diet rich in fruit and vegetables encouraging bacterial diversity, which improves health. We benefit from a symbiotic relationship with nature, even at the microscopic level.

## Adverse childhood experiences

Our social development influences our health as much as our physical environment. Self-esteem, sense of meaning, relationships and social capital all affect our health, and any lack of these, particularly in our formative years, worsens health. *Adverse childhood experiences* (ACEs) are recognised to be strongly linked to adverse health outcomes later in life. ACEs are potentially traumatic experiences during formative years, such as the experience of violence, abuse or neglect (Table 2.6). Unstable parenting is a significant risk, especially when combined with a lack of alternative adult role models. Problematic drug or alcohol use, and forensic or mental health problems

*Table 2.6* Adverse childhood experiences

| | |
|---|---|
| Emotional abuse | Humiliation, bullying or fear of being hurt by a household adult |
| Physical abuse | Physical violence leaving a mark or injury |
| Sexual abuse | Being touched or interfered with sexually by an adult or person at least five years older |
| Emotional neglect | Feeling unloved or unimportant |
| Physical neglect | Being malnourished or neglected |
| Separation | Parental separation or divorce |
| Household violence | Domestic violence in the household |
| Household substance abuse | Problematic alcohol or drug use in the household |
| Household mental illness | Mental illness or suicide in a household member |
| Household incarceration | Imprisonment of a household member |

within the household are also damaging, causing *traumatic toxic stress*. This differs from tolerable stress in which difficulties are buffered by adaptation with the help of caring adults.

The first identification of the impact of ACEs developed from the recognition that adults attending an obesity clinic had high rates of childhood abuse (Vincent Felitti).[41] Obesity had become a solution; gaining weight offered protection against unwanted sexual attention.[42] Smoking, drug or alcohol use may protect in the short term, by helping to regulate mood, but these have harmful outcomes over the longer term. ACEs lead to impairment of social, emotional and cognitive development, causing unhealthy behaviours that contribute to early morbidity and mortality.

In England, almost one in two people has at least one ACE, while one in fourteen people has four or more.[43] There is a strong link between ACEs and deprivation, and multiple ACEs are associated with far poorer health outcomes, especially violence, problematic alcohol/drug use, sexual risk taking and poor mental health.[44] A male with six ACEs is forty-six times more likely to use intravenous drugs than someone with no ACEs, drugs offering a way to relieve distress. Having four ACEs gives an almost three-fold increased risk of being diagnosed with a major disease below the age of seventy.

Other experiences have been suggested in addition to the original list of ten ACEs. Traumatic loss of a loved one, frequent relocations, a life-threatening illness, and exposure to war, terrorism and natural disasters all destabilise childhood.[45] Child poverty has the strongest link to adverse outcomes, as higher incomes protect against the damage from factors such as separation or incarceration. The combination of poverty and parental mental health problems brings the highest risk of poor outcomes.[46]

Multiple less severe experiences may also add up to significant cumulative damage. Not feeling safe is a potent stressor for situations that might otherwise be manageable. The constancy of microaggressions experienced by people in marginalised groups worsens outcomes. Coping involves both dealing with the problem causing distress and managing the emotion that arises.

## Physiology of trauma

The physiological processes underlying the damage caused by trauma are clear. *Allostatic load* refers to the degenerative changes to a body as a result of exposure to repeated or chronic stress, allostasis meaning 'achieving stability through change'. The pathophysiological effects of chronic exposure to stress hormones and overdrive of the sympathetic nervous system cause increased inflammation and altered adaptations to stress.[47] Inflammation is linked with many diseases, including dementia and heart disease. Even accounting for weight, smoking and other risk factors, the inflammatory marker C-reactive protein is higher in more deprived populations.[48]

Allostatic load leads to worsened health outcomes in people of minority ethnicity. Racism is bad for health, not just for those being discriminated against but also those who hold racist views. Belief in differing ability between ethnicities worsens mortality in both Black and white Americans.[49] Black people in the USA have shorter life expectancy, which was promoted as evidence to justify *biological determinism*, the idea of genetic inferiority which bred oppression and eugenics. Careful work over a century ago by William Du Bois, a sociologist and activist, showed instead that socioeconomic factors were responsible for the difference, and that white people in poverty had a similar increase in mortality.[50]

Abnormalities in cortisol levels from traumatic toxic stress increase the risk of both infection and autoimmune conditions. Remodelling in areas of the brain such as the amygdala and prefrontal cortex, which regulate emotions, increases impulsive behaviour.[51] ACEs alter the way genes are expressed. Known as *epigenetic* changes, the DNA code (genotype) stays the same, but the expression (phenotype) alters, allowing a rapid response to changes in the environment. These epigenetic changes have even been shown in utero in response to maternal hardship.

ACEs are linked with cellular ageing. *Telomeres* are a protective 'cap' at the end of chromosomes, which shortens as cells age, limiting the number of possible cell divisions. Stress prematurely ages cells, with shorter telomere lengths correlating with ACEs, especially early exposure and physical neglect.[52] Shortened telomeres can even be heritable by children, the effects of traumatic experiences crossing generations. These transgenerational effects can be seen in the lower birth weights of babies born to Black American mothers. Lower birth weights are associated with a variety of poor outcomes including high blood pressure and metabolic risk factors for cardiovascular disease such as diabetes and high cholesterol. Driven by structural inequality and discrimination, damage mediated through epigenetic changes spreads the effects of toxic stress across generations.[53]

The risk of focusing on ACEs is that of pathologising individuals, while losing sight of the structural problems that led to these situations. We see the smoke of unhealthy behaviours, but miss the fire of adversity causing those behaviours. The link between ACEs and poor health outcomes is clear. Breaking this cycle for future generations means both preventing ACEs and reducing the associated trauma.

Asking about ACEs can be daunting. Fear of having to deal with disclosures, coupled with the perception of risk that comes from dealing with people who are distressed, means emotional concerns are often minimised during consultations. Explaining that ACEs can sometimes be associated with symptom clusters can open up conversations that avoid retraumatising. Reactions to adversity vary significantly, so the phrase 'potentially traumatic events' is more accessible. There are concerns that asking about ACEs is unethical without offering treatments,[54] though interventions that reduce the impact of these experiences are available. It is important not to focus purely on an ACE score, and it should not be used to prioritise interventions. While there is not yet evidence that screening for ACEs improves outcomes, clinicians asking about ACEs seems to be acceptable to patients, although discussion in a therapeutic environment takes time and understanding.[55]

Effective interventions are available for both targeted and wider groups.[56] These work to improve attachment, which is crucial for healthy development in early years. The highest returns come from intervening at the earliest possible stage.[57] Parenting support programmes and learning social and emotional skills at school should be available universally. Perinatal mental health screening and asking about intimate partner violence during pregnancy identifies those who would benefit from effective treatments such as cognitive behavioural therapy (CBT). More targeted interventions offered to children and parents help those at risk from ACEs.

There is good evidence for parenting classes such as Incredible Years and Triple P. The targeted group programme Empowering Parents, Empowering Communities for preschool children is cheap (less than £100 per person) and has shown short-term positive impacts on child outcomes. The Family Nurse Partnership home-visiting programme teaches parenting skills to expectant mothers. The relationship between client and nurse is an important part of the process, and has positive long-term impacts across a range of outcomes for the child. The costs (over £2,000 per participant) are far less significant when weighed against the long-term health sequelae of adverse experiences. Investing in childcare returns nearly five times the investment.[58] Rebuilding trust that has been eroded by multiple ACEs is the common ingredient in effective interventions. Community-based models that encourage these supportive relationships rebuild trust and social identity.

*Table 2.7* Common unmet psychological needs[a]

| | |
|---|---|
| Self esteem | Appraisal of one's own worth, which should be sufficient but not excessive |
| Competence | Feeling in control of circumstances and capable of solving problems |
| Autonomy | Feeling in control of own behaviour |
| Relatedness | Being appreciated by other people |
| Security | Living without fear of being harmed |

Note:
a  Watts B, Young Foundation (London E. *Sinking & Swimming: Understanding Britain's Unmet Needs*. The Young Foundation; 2009). https://youngfoundation.org/wp-content/uploads/2012/10/Sinking-and-swimming.pdf

### Trauma-informed communities

The recognition that the effects of childhood trauma can show in patterns of adult behaviour have led to the development of trauma-informed approaches. These consider symptoms as signals that something is amiss, which moves the focus from 'what is wrong with you?' to 'what happened to you?' Caregivers and others need to be aware of how their actions can perpetuate trauma. People feeling powerless may be cautious in situations where a power imbalance may persist, precipitating hyperalert states which may not be recognised or understood by those around them. For example, someone with previous traumatic experience may fear being trapped in a room. Closing a door behind that person may trigger panic or similar reactions, without necessarily a recognition of the cause. This embodiment of fear can lead to disconnected or hypervigilant states.

*Dissociation* describes a separation of sensory experience from a sense of identity. Separating one's sense of self from a traumatic experience allows these events to appear to happen to someone else, and is a creative way children in particular use to compartmentalise and cope with such experiences. Using this as a defence mechanism for childhood traumata can lead to ongoing dissociation as a coping strategy in adulthood. This may cause symptoms such as depersonalisation, a detachment from sense of self, or derealisation, detachment from the surrounding environment. This disconnection and diminished awareness of emotions or thoughts is a protective strategy, but sustaining these avoidant behaviours can lead to problematic sexual behaviour, food, drug or alcohol use and self-injury.

Dissociation occurs along a continuum from ordinary daydreaming to pathological states where function or behaviour is impacted. We all dissociate, for around 10 per cent of the day.[59] When used as a defence mechanism for unendurable events, arranging these highly emotional sensations into memory is difficult. This protects us by making recalling events harder, but fragments of these emotional states can continue to intrude into consciousness outside of the original context. In the past, persistent dissociation would have been diagnosed as witchcraft,[60] hysteria or schizophrenia, but is now recognised as a response to trauma, in part due to understanding symptoms in veterans and survivors of conflict. Diagnoses increasingly reflect the effects of post-traumatic stress and complex emotional trauma, but still locate the problem as being with the individual rather than from the systemic effects of inequity and oppression.

Being trauma-informed seeks to understand the reasons underlying behaviour, and offers helpful explanations for how to avoid responding to a heightened emotional state in the same manner. What happened may not be our business, but understanding that what we are seeing may be the repercussions of past experiences helps adapt responses to be more helpful. Finding ways to restore control to the individual helps defuse threatening situations. This applies both to those working with individuals in heightened emotional states and more widely, to all of us dealing with other people. Better awareness of the impact of ACEs is important, particularly for those who work with others. Providing training on ACEs[61] facilitates a more widespread uptake of learning, potentially leading to a whole town approach of a trauma-informed community.

## Resilience

Resilience, the ability to adapt to adverse circumstances, is a simplistic solution to complex problems. Focusing on resilience diverts any need for system change by identifying the problem as being with individuals, who must internalise a view of their deficit and learn to adapt to a situation. While it may be convenient for those who benefit from the status quo to suggest that problems are moral failings and not a maladaptive or malign system, this view of resilience exists to support existing power structures rather than individuals.

Resilience is usually latent, becoming apparent at times of adversity. Some individuals have good outcomes despite highly adverse circumstances, showing how important protective factors can be. Single-event trauma and chronic adversity provoke different responses, prompting the terms *emergent resilience* as a response to chronic adversity and *minimal-impact resilience* to describe that to an acute life event.[62] This fits with the diagnostic labels of complex post-traumatic stress disorder (PTSD) from chronic exposure to stress, and PTSD in response to a single traumatic event. The chronicity of exposure is more significant than the circumstances; ongoing parental conflict is more damaging than the loss of a parent.[63]

The word *resilience* derives from the Latin *resalire*, meaning 'to spring back'. Bad days happen to all of us, when we have to cope with difficult circumstances, but most people bounce back from these, most of the time. For some, the recovery does not happen, and an individual enters a more passive state of ongoing negative emotion. A shift into depression usually entails withdrawal, whether from food, companionship, work or pastimes. Sleep disturbance in particular is a sensitive predictor of depression. Early morning wakening is the most specific symptom of depression. Low mood triggers anxieties that resurface during restless nights, perpetuating a cycle of early waking and fatigue. Hypervigilance and the time needed to process emotions disturb night-time rest, leading to a vicious cycle of chronic tiredness, with a lack of refreshing sleep reinforcing low mood the following day. Unrefreshing sleep is associated with a variety of conditions including chronic pain and mental health problems.[64]

Being able to consider alternative explanations for events is a particular skill, associated with empathy, allowing a flexible narrative around circumstances. Resilience is very strongly associated with networks of support, even ordinary day-to-day interactions increasing the feeling of connectedness. Finding the meaning in events is an important skill in developing resilience, as hopelessness and despair are potent forces causing distress. Despite the

*Table 2.8* Factors increasing resilience ('ordinary magic', Ann Masten)[a]

| Attachment | Positive attachments |
|---|---|
| | Positive nurturing relationships with competent adults |
| | Supportive friends |
| Competences | Intellectual skills |
| | Self-regulation skills, executive functions allowing self-control |
| Socio-cultural | Bonds to prosocial organisations such as schools |
| | Community bonds supporting families |
| | Cultural support |
| Positive self-perceptions | Meaning in life, encompassing faith and hopelessness |

Note:
a  Masten AS. Ordinary magic: lessons from research on resilience in human development. *Educ Can.* 2009;49:28–32.

secularisation of society, attributing events to a higher power remains culturally embedded.

Being in good mental health has other beneficial effects. Positive emotions widen our repertoires of thought-action ('broaden-and-build', Barbara Fredrickson).[65] Feelings such as pride or love expand our behaviours, increasing our resources. Negative emotions instead tend to inspire narrow 'fight or flight' reactions. A positive emotion such as joy is associated with play, which builds skills. The attachments love inspires are strongly protective. Interest leads to exploration, while contentment is a low-arousal, positive emotion which allows reflection and a mindful broadening of views.

The presence of these protective factors does not guarantee resilience, especially where other circumstances interact. Black youths in America show higher allostatic load, as measured by stress hormones and physiological parameters, even in the presence of high psychosocial competence and low levels of adjustment problems.[66] Positive factors and adaptive coping strategies may not be enough to override systemic discrimination, especially at the intersection of multiple forms of marginalisation, where the effects of injustice become amplified.

Resilience is a facet of communities as well as individuals. Community resilience is 'the ability of social groups to withstand and recover from unfavourable circumstances'.[67] Effective leadership inspires other leaders and encourages strengths already within the team. Mutual trust and deep social networks protect and promote health and wellbeing. Diversity makes a community more adaptive, and thus less vulnerable to future threats.

Resilience can be quantified using the Resilience Measure, with versions available for youths and adults.[68] Strong resilience scores reflect sources of support, skills, sense of belonging and being able to identify trusted role models, all of which protect from the damage of exposure to ACEs.[69]

Interventions to improve resilience work by reducing exposure to risk, lessening the damage from the interaction of risk factors and creating the circumstances and opportunity for change.[70] Having access to a trusted adult other than a parent or primary caregiver in childhood is protective, providing alternative routes for help. Intergenerational bonds are important, especially between girls and other female family members, and can be a strong buffer in adversity. Young people benefit from mentors who offer positive models of adulthood. Encouraging adolescents to take up social roles promotes competence, and the ability to manage these roles predicts ability to cope. Supportive and understanding employers can change lives. Services that are overly cautious in avoiding any perceived risk miss the role of adversity in creating resilience. Stresses are needed to build strength.

Many of the factors that influence our health are outside the reach of current healthcare provision. These factors are amenable to intervention, but need approaching in a different way. Building social capital and cohesion improves resilience and protects against the damage caused by inequality and marginalisation. These determinants of health happen in our communities, and communities are the best place to address them.

## Notes

Links and additional resources for this chapter can be found at www.communityhealth. uk/2-health-and-its-determinants

1　WHO Centre for Health Development (Kobe, Japan). *A Glossary of Terms for Community Health Care and Services for Older Persons*; 2004. https://apps.who. int/iris/handle/10665/68896
2　Carel HH. Illness, phenomenology, and philosophical method. *Theor Med Bioeth*. 2013;34(4):345–357. doi:10.1007/s11017-013-9265-1.
3　Gadamer HG. *The Enigma of Health*. Polity Press; 1996.
4　Ventriglio A, Torales J, Bhugra D. Disease versus illness: what do clinicians need to know? *Int J Soc Psychiatry*. 2017;63(1):3–4. doi:10.1177/0020764016658677.
5　Cassell EJ. *The Healer's Art: A New Approach to the Doctor-Patient Relationship*. Penguin Books; 1978.
6　Toombs SK. The temporality of illness: four levels of experience. *Theor Med*. 1990;11(3):227–241. doi:10.1007/BF00489832.
7　Chrisman NJ. The health seeking process: an approach to the natural history of illness. *Cult Med Psychiatry*. 1977;1(4):351–377. doi:10.1007/BF00116243.
8　Bar-Haim S. 'The Drug Doctor': Michael Balint and the revival of general practice in postwar Britain. *Hist Workshop J*. 2018;86:114–132. doi:10.1093/hwj/ dby017.
9　Balestra C, Boarini R, Tosetto E. What matters most to people? Evidence from the OECD Better Life Index users' responses. *Soc Indic Res*. 2018;136(3):907–930. doi:10.1007/s11205-016-1538-4.
10　Mackenbach JP. Politics is nothing but medicine at a larger scale: reflections on public health's biggest idea. *J Epidemiol Community Health*. 2009;63(3):181–184. doi:10.1136/jech.2008.077032.
11　Yusuf S, Joseph P, Rangarajan S, et al. Modifiable risk factors, cardiovascular disease, and mortality in 155 722 individuals from 21 high-income, middle-income, and low-income countries (PURE): a prospective cohort study. *The Lancet*. 2020;395(10226):795–808. doi:10.1016/S0140-6736(19)32008-2.
12　Marmot, Michael, Allen, Jessica, Goldblatt, Peter, et al. *Fair Society, Healthy Lives: The Marmot Review*. UCL; 2010. https://www.instituteofhealthequity.org/ resources-reports/fair-society-healthy-lives-the-marmot-review

13  Public Health England. *Psychosis Data Report: Describing Variation in Numbers of People with Psychosis and Their Access to Care in England.* Public Health England; 2016:77. https://assets.publishing.service.gov.uk/government/uploads/system/uploads/attachment_data/file/774680/Psychosis_data_report.pdf

14  See note 12.

15  Wilkinson RG. Socioeconomic determinants of health: health inequalities: relative or absolute material standards? *BMJ.* 1997;314(7080):591–591. doi:10.1136/bmj.314.7080.591.

16  Fitzpatrick S, Bramley G, Blenkinsopp J, et al. *Destitution in the UK.* Joseph Rowntree Foundation; 2020. https://www.jrf.org.uk/report/destitution-uk-2020

17  Alston, Philip. *Statement on Visit to the United Kingdom, by Professor Philip Alston, United Nations Special Rapporteur on Extreme Poverty and Human Rights*; 2018. https://www.ohchr.org/sites/default/files/Documents/Issues/Poverty/EOM_GB_16Nov2018.pdf

18  Barry, Andrea, Brook, Paul, Cebula, Carla, et al. *UK Poverty 2022.* Joseph Rowntree Foundation; 2022. https://www.jrf.org.uk/report/uk-poverty-2022

19  Scott, Courtney, Sutherland, Jennifer, Taylor, Anna. *Affordability of the UK's Eatwell Guide.* The Food Foundation; 2018. https://foodfoundation.org.uk/publication/affordability-uks-eatwell-guide

20  Macdonald L, Olsen JR, Shortt NK, Ellaway A. Do 'environmental bads' such as alcohol, fast food, tobacco, and gambling outlets cluster and co-locate in more deprived areas in Glasgow? *Health Place.* 2018;51:224–231. doi:10.1016/j.healthplace.2018.04.008.

21  QIntervention is a cardiovascular risk calculator, based on real time risk data, which shows the effects of changing risk factors such as stopping smoking or taking a statin. QIntervention. https://qintervention.org/

22  Cookson R, Propper C, Asaria M, Raine R. Socio-economic inequalities in health care in England. *Fisc Stud.* 2016;37(3-4):371–403. doi:10.1111/j.1475-5890.2016.12109.

23  Tudor Hart J. The inverse care law. *The Lancet.* 1971;297(7696):405–412. doi:10.1016/S0140-6736(71)92410-X.

24  Marmot M, Allen J, Boyce T, Goldblatt P, Morrison J. *Health Equity in England: The Marmot Report 10 Years On.* Institute of Health Equity; 2020:172.

25  Wilkinson RG, Pickett K. *The Spirit Level: Why Equality Is Better for Everyone.* Penguin Books; 2010.

26  Alesina, Alberto, Rodrik, Dani. *Distributive Politics and Economic Growth.* National Bureau of Economic Research; 1991:54. https://www.nber.org/papers/w3668

27  Each standard deviation reduction in income inequality increases GDP by 8.2 per cent after a generation. Birdsall N, Ross D, Sabot R. Inequality and growth reconsidered: lessons from East Asia. *World Bank Econ Rev.* 1995;9(3):477–508. doi:10.1093/wber/9.3.477.

28  Kennedy BP, Kawachi I, Prothrow-Stith D. Income distribution and mortality: cross sectional ecological study of the Robin Hood index in the United States. *BMJ.* 1996;312(7037):1004–1007. doi:10.1136/bmj.312.7037.1004.

29  See note 12.

30  Rodgers GB. Income and inequality as determinants of mortality: an international cross-section analysis. *Popul Stud.* 1979;33(2):343–351. doi:10.1080/00324728.1979.10410449.

31  See note 15.

32  Kaplan GA, Pamuk ER, Lynch JW, Cohen RD, Balfour JL. Inequality in income and mortality in the United States: analysis of mortality and potential pathways. *BMJ.* 1996;312(7037):999–1003. doi:10.1136/bmj.312.7037.999.

33  Putnam RD, Leonardi R, Nanetti R. *Making Democracy Work: Civic Traditions in Modern Italy.* Princeton University Press; 1993.

34  See note 15.

35 Kennedy, Bruce, Kawachi, Ichiro, 10.1136/bmj.312.7037.1004. Important correction to Income distribution and mortality: cross sectional ecological study of the Robin Hood index in the United States. *BMJ.* 1996;312(7040):1194–1194. doi:10.1136/bmj.312.7040.1194.

36 Barker D. The origins of the developmental origins theory. *J Intern Med.* 2007;261(5):412–417. doi:10.1111/j.1365-2796.2007.01809.x.

37 Robertson RC, Manges AR, Finlay BB. The human microbiome and child growth; first 1000 days and beyond. *Trends Microbiol.* 2019;27(2):131–147. doi:10.1016/j.tim.2018.09.008.

38 O'Mahony S, Clarke G, Borre Y, Dinan T, Cryan J. Serotonin, tryptophan metabolism and the brain-gut-microbiome axis. *Behav Brain Res.* 2015;277:32–48. doi:10.1016/j.bbr.2014.07.027.

39 Trasande L, Blustein J, Liu M, Corwin E, Cox LM, Blaser MJ. Infant antibiotic exposures and early-life body mass. *Int J Obes.* 2013;37(1):16–23. doi:10.1038/ijo.2012.132.

40 Gilbert JA, Blaser MJ, Caporaso JG, Jansson JK, Lynch SV, Knight R. Current understanding of the human microbiome. *Nat Med.* 2018;24(4):392–400. doi:10.1038/nm.4517.

41 Felitti VJ. Relationship of childhood abuse and household dysfunction to many of the leading causes of death in adults: the adverse childhood experiences (ACE) study. *Am J Prev Med.* 1998;14(2):245–258. doi:10.1016/S0749-3797(98)00017-8.

42 Felitti VJ. The relation between adverse childhood experiences and adult health: turning gold into lead. *Perm J.* 2002;6(1):44–47. doi:10.7812/TPP/02.994.

43 Bellis MA, Hughes K, Leckenby N, Hardcastle KA, Perkins C, Lowey H. Measuring mortality and the burden of adult disease associated with adverse childhood experiences in England: a national survey. *J Public Health.* 2014;37(3):445–454. doi:10.1093/pubmed/fdu065.

44 Hughes K, Bellis MA, Hardcastle KA, et al. The effect of multiple adverse childhood experiences on health: a systematic review and meta-analysis. *Lancet Public Health.* 2017;2(8):e356–e366. doi:10.1016/S2468-2667(17)30118-4.

45 Oral R, Ramirez M, Coohey C, et al. Adverse childhood experiences and trauma informed care: the future of health care. *Pediatr Res.* 2016;79(1):227–233. doi:10.1038/pr.2015.197.

46 Lanier P, Maguire-Jack K, Lombardi B, Frey J, Rose RA. Adverse childhood experiences and child health outcomes: comparing cumulative risk and latent class approaches. *Matern Child Health J.* 2018;22(3):288–297. doi:10.1007/s10995-017-2365-1.

47 McEwen BS. Physiology and neurobiology of stress and adaptation: central role of the brain. *Physiol Rev.* 2007;87(3):873–904. doi:10.1152/physrev.00041.2006.

48 Davillas A, Benzeval M, Kumari M. Socio-economic inequalities in C-reactive protein and fibrinogen across the adult age span: findings from understanding society. *Sci Rep.* 2017;7(1):2641. doi:10.1038/s41598-017-02888-6.

49 Kennedy BP, Kawachi I, Lochner K, Jones C, Prothrow-Stith D. (Dis)respect and black mortality. *Ethn Dis.* 1997;7(3):207–214.

50 White K. The sustaining relevance of W. E. B. Du Bois to health disparities research. *Bois Rev Soc Sci Res Race.* 2011;8(1):285–293. doi:10.1017/S1742058X11000233.

51 See note 47.

52 Lang J, McKie J, Smith H, et al. Adverse childhood experiences, epigenetics and telomere length variation in childhood and beyond: a systematic review of the literature. *Eur Child Adolesc Psychiatry.* 2020;29(10):1329–1338. doi:10.1007/s00787-019-01329-1.

53 Kuzawa CW, Sweet E. Epigenetics and the embodiment of race: developmental origins of US racial disparities in cardiovascular health. *Am J Hum Biol.* 2009;21(1):2–15. doi:10.1002/ajhb.20822.

54 Finkelhor D. Screening for adverse childhood experiences (ACEs): cautions and suggestions. *Child Abuse Negl.* 2018;85:174–179. doi:10.1016/j.chiabu.2017.07.016.

55 Asmussen K, Fischer F, Drayton E, McBride T. *Adverse Childhood Experiences: What We Know, What We Don't Know, and What Should Happen Next.* Early Intervention Foundation; 2020. https://www.eif.org.uk/report/adverse-childhood-experiences-what-we-know-what-we-dont-know-and-what-should-happen-next

56 EIF. Early Intervention Federation Guidebook. Published March 20, 2017. https://guidebook.eif.org.uk/home/

57 The 'Heckman curve' is a visualisation of how the earliest investments in children bring the biggest rewards. Heckman JJ. Skill formation and the economics of investing in disadvantaged children. *Science.* 2006;312(5782):1900–1902. doi:10.1126/science.1128898.

58 Aked, Jody, Steuer, Nicola, Lawlor, Eilis, Spratt, Stephen. *Backing the Future: Why Investing in Children Is Good for Us All.* New Economics Foundation; 2009. https://neweconomics.org/2009/09/backing-the-future

59 Diseth TH. Dissociation in children and adolescents as reaction to trauma – an overview of conceptual issues and neurobiological factors. *Nord J Psychiatry.* 2005;59(2):79–91. doi:10.1080/08039480510022963.

60 Harding, Keir. Diagnosing borderline personality disorder: a 21st century witch hunt. Beam Consultancy. Published October 21, 2020. https://www.beamconsultancy.co.uk/the-blog/2020/10/21/diagnosing-borderline-personality-disorder-a-21stnbspcentury-witch-hunt

61 For example, ACEs online learning. https://www.acesonlinelearning.com

62 Bonanno GA, Diminich ED. Annual research review: positive adjustment to adversity: trajectories of minimal-impact resilience and emergent resilience. *J Child Psychol Psychiatry.* 2012;54(4):378–401. doi:10.1111/jcpp.12021.

63 Turk J, Graham PJ, Verhulst FC, Graham PJ. *Child and Adolescent Psychiatry: A Developmental Approach.* 4th ed. Oxford University Press; 2007.

64 Moldofsky H. Sleep and pain. *Sleep Med Rev.* 2001;5(5):385–396. doi:10.1053/smrv.2001.0179.

65 Fredrickson BL. What good are positive emotions? *Rev Gen Psychol J Div 1 Am Psychol Assoc.* 1998;2(3):300–319. doi:10.1037/1089-2680.2.3.300.

66 Brody GH, Yu T, Chen E, Miller GE, Kogan SM, Beach SRH. Is resilience only skin deep?: rural African Americans' socioeconomic status–related risk and competence in preadolescence and psychological adjustment and allostatic load at age 19. *Psychol Sci.* 2013;24(7):1285–1293. doi:10.1177/0956797612471954.

67 World Health Organization. *Strengthening Resilience: A Priority Shared by Health 2020 and the Sustainable Development Goals*; 2017. https://www.euro.who.int/__data/assets/pdf_file/0005/351284/resilience-report-20171004-h1635.pdf

68 Child and Youth Resilience Measure & Adult Resilience Measure. https://cyrm.resilienceresearch.org/

69 See note 44.

70 Newman T, University of Exeter. Centre for Evidence-Based Social Services (GB). *Promoting resilience: a review of effective strategies for child care services*; 2002. https://www.cumbria.gov.uk/eLibrary/Content/Internet/537/6942/6944/6954/42191163412.pdf Notes and links for this chapter can be found at communityhealth.uk/2-health-and-its-determinants

# 3  Disorders of society

The downstream effects of inequality and discrimination manifest in poorer physical and mental health across populations. Poverty, societal dysfunction and the impacts of childhood adversity all lead to worse health outcomes. The poor health these cause leads to expensive welfare and healthcare costs. Healthcare institutions end up managing the health impacts of these determinants of our health, but intervening earlier would reduce the damage and financial cost.

## Loneliness

Lack of human companionship is a major risk factor for illness, but loneliness is under-recognised both in our society and within healthcare. Those who are most isolated are twice as likely to die as those with extensive contacts.[1] Part of the reason loneliness is hidden is mathematical; lonely people have few connections, so not many people know someone who is lonely. Loneliness carries a stigma, hiding in and out of sight, social faces kept in a jar by the door.

Loneliness is a subjective, unwelcome feeling of lack of companionship, which happens when there is a mismatch between the quantity and quality of social relationships that we have and those that we would like. While loneliness is subjective, social isolation describes a more objective lack of social contacts. We can be isolated but not lonely, or lonely in a crowd. Loneliness has both emotional and social components, related to lack of attachment figures or social networks respectively. Loneliness raises sensitivity to threats, generating defensive behaviours including rejecting others, which lessens short-term distress but perpetuates the problem in the longer term.[2] Our need to be among others is an evolutionary adaptation that, by bringing us back to family or tribe, helped our survival as a species.

It is common to have times in our lives when our social contacts are much reduced, usually around times of loss or transition such as moving or changing school or job. These changes leave us isolated, triggering a 'reaffiliation motive' to connect with others.[3] Some people are less able to rebuild connections, leading to more persistent loneliness. Reconnection fails, and negative cognitive biases precipitate further social withdrawal, reinforcing ongoing

DOI: 10.4324/9781003391784-4

*Table 3.1* Loneliness

| | |
|---|---|
| Mortality | The risk of dying increases for the most lonely compared to those with extensive contacts: 2.3 higher in men, 2.8 higher in women.[a] Lonely older adults are twice as likely to die within six years as the least lonely.[b] |
| Cost | Loneliness costs the UK £9,900 per person annually predominantly due to negative effects on wellbeing,[c] with a total annual cost to employers of £2.5 bn.[d] |

Notes:

a  Berkman L, Syme SL. Social networks, host resistance and mortality: A nine-year follow-up study of Alameda County residents. *Am J Epidemiol.* 1979;109(2):186-204. doi:10.1093/oxfordjournals.aje.a112674

b  Luo Y, Hawkley LC, Waite LJ, Cacioppo JT. Loneliness, health, and mortality in old age: A national longitudinal study. *Soc Sci Med.* 2012;74(6):907-914. doi:10.1016/j.socscimed.2011.11.028

c  Peytrignet, Sebastien, Garforth-Bles, Simon, Keohane, Kieran. *Loneliness Monetisation Report.* Department for Digital, Culture, Media & Sport; 2020. https://www.gov.uk/government/publications/loneliness-monetisation-report

d  Qualter, Pamela. *Tackling Loneliness Evidence Review: Main Report.* Dept for Digital, Culture, Media and Sport, UK Government; 2022. https://www.gov.uk/government/publications/tackling-loneliness-evidence-review/tackling-loneliness-evidence-review-full-report

loneliness. Avoiding contacts protects against the chance of rejection, while the lost opportunities to maintain social skills perpetuate a state of disconnection, so loneliness becomes self-sustaining.

Nine million adults in the UK are often or always lonely,[4] television the main companion for many. There is a perception that loneliness is a condition affecting older people, but younger people are most likely to report feeling lonely.[5] The development of independence coupled with peer group expectations make this an age of transition, where social connections are not always those desired. Loneliness in middle childhood (from eight to eleven years) carries the most significant impact into later life.[6] Other adverse factors, such as victimisation and family conflict, contribute to loneliness in children and young people.[7] This leaves longer term health problems; cardiovascular disease markers increase according to the degree of isolation in childhood.[8]

People in marginalised groups are at higher risk of loneliness, with migrants and people of minority ethnicity, gender and sexuality all at increased risk. A built environment poorly adapted to the needs of disabled people limits opportunities for interactions. Hearing impairments shut people out of conversations, more so now when face coverings are needed. Other correlates for loneliness are disability, caring roles, not being in employment, being single, widowed or living alone and lacking trust in others locally. While some isolated jobs such as farming carry increased risk, loneliness is associated more with urban and deprived areas than rural ones.

For younger people, quantity seems to be an important factor in social relationships, while quality is more important for older people.[9] Married people are less likely to be lonely, but it is the quality of a marriage that protects most against loneliness. Those who feel a sense of belonging to their neighbourhood and have higher trust in neighbours feel less lonely.[10]

Workplace loneliness affects a third of employees juggling work and caring roles.[11] Loneliness is more common in individualist societies,[12] and corporate cultures that emphasise competition and individualism also exacerbate loneliness. Remote working and a gig economy favouring temporary contracts are leading to greater workplace loneliness.

Loneliness worsens our health, and is associated with a range of conditions including asthma, arthritis, migraine, tinnitus, alcohol use and mental health problems in young people.[13] People who are lonely are twice as likely to die following cardiac bypass surgery.[14] Married people, especially men, have lower mortality than those who are single, divorced or widowed.[15] Isolation actually reduces the likelihood of migraine, osteoarthritis and alcohol problems, but increases the risk of mental health conditions. Those who are least socially integrated have more than four times as many colds, even after accounting for better immunity in those with more contacts.[16]

Our bodies show physiological changes due to loneliness, with worse sleep and lower sleep efficiency (time spent asleep vs time wanting to be asleep).[17] This increases sympathetic tone and evening cortisol levels, reducing tolerance to glucose which causes damaging spikes of blood sugar. This is a type of stress response, the common link being feeling unsafe. Loneliness makes perceived environmental threats more potent and the external world more sinister, reinforcing any tendency to withdraw. People who are less integrated are less likely to be encouraged to look after themselves and seek help when needed, reinforcing the health impacts of loneliness.

Improving our social relationships halves our risk of dying.[18] Joining a group carries the same reduction in mortality as stopping smoking.[19] Group-based interventions for older people that promote peer support and social integration improve wellbeing and increase new friends, but this may not be enough to improve loneliness scores.[20] There is also a need to address negative thinking patterns which perpetuate a state of loneliness. Interventions that build social and emotional skills are effective, as are those that encourage learning a new hobby.[21] Using technology to facilitate intergenerational conversations remotely reduces loneliness in older people.[22] Providing personalised proactive support to increase social connections, with the aim of boosting resilience and self-esteem, saves money and reduces loneliness scores.[23] The most effective interventions address unhelpful social cognition[24] along with improving social skills, support and opportunities for contact.

There is a risk that loneliness becomes medicalised into a disease to be treated. Using healthcare as the access point for people who are lonely undermines community approaches. Addressing loneliness in our communities comes from creating an accessible and welcoming society that encourages connections.

*Table 3.2* Measuring loneliness and isolation

| | |
|---|---|
| Direct question | 'How often do you feel lonely?' |
| Indirect questions | The three item UCLA Loneliness scale records how often one feels lacking companionship, feeling left out, or feeling isolated from others |
| Other measures | De Jong Gierveld Scale for Loneliness (6 and 11 question versions) |
| | Social Isolation score:[a] |
| | One point for each of the following, to a maximum score of five, higher scores representing more isolation: |
| | • Unmarried / not cohabitating |
| | • Less than monthly contact with one's children |
| | • Less than monthly contact with other family members |
| | • Less than monthly contact with friends |
| | • Not participating in organisations / social groups |

Note:
a Steptoe A, Shankar A, Demakakos P, Wardle J. Social isolation, loneliness, and all-cause mortality in older men and women. *Proc Natl Acad Sci.* 2013;110(15):5797-5801. doi:10.1073/pnas.1219686110

## Dementia

Dementia is an increasingly common condition, straddling mental and physical health. Diagnosis rates in the UK have more than doubled in the decade up to 2020,[25] as improvements in life expectancy mean more people survive to experience degenerative conditions in later life. Dementia comprises far more than just memory loss, with varying difficulties across speech, vision, spatial reasoning and carrying out the activities of daily life.

Dementia, depression and loneliness are strongly linked. Even after controlling for depression, loneliness remains an independent risk factor doubling the risk of dementia.[26] Health-damaging behaviours and a disengagement from self-care cause some of the risk. Lack of social contact causes nerve damage, both directly and by inhibiting cellular repair. Shortened telomeres, limiting the ability of cells to regenerate, are seen in both loneliness and dementia. The cellular burden is similar to that from chronic stress, with persistent inflammation and stress hormone release reducing interconnections between nerves.[27]

Lonely people lay down more than seven times as much amyloid in the brain,[28] amyloid being folded sheets of protein deposited abnormally within brain tissue associated with Alzheimer's disease. This change is not seen in dementia due to vascular disease, suggesting loneliness may predispose specifically to the pathological changes of Alzheimer's.[29] These changes are preventable and even reversible ('rementia'),[30] amenable to interventions that reduce loneliness and stress. Increased social participation reduces the chance of Alzheimer's disease; preventing dementia happens at community level.

Dementia is an illness defined most during interactions with others. The predominant loss in dementia is a sense of personhood, due to the prevalent view of dementia that focuses on deficits and misses the abilities that people with dementia retain (Figure 3.1). This pathologising view ignores the need

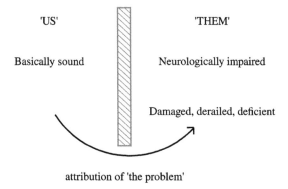

*Figure 3.1* Personhood in dementia.

Kitwood T, Bredin K. Towards a Theory of Dementia Care: Personhood and Well-being. *Ageing Soc.* 1992;12(03):269-287. doi:10.1017/S0144686X0000502X.

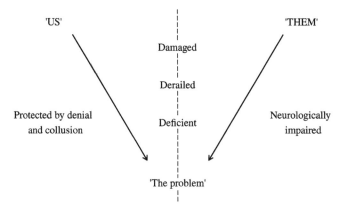

*Figure 3.2* Shared solutions.

Kitwood T, Bredin K. Towards a Theory of Dementia Care: Personhood and Well-being. *Ageing Soc.* 1992;12(03):269-287. doi:10.1017/S0144686X0000502X.

for systemic changes by relocating the problem to the individual, an 'othering' that occurs across many other health conditions as well.

People living even with severe dementia show many behaviours that confirm their personhood in relation to others: asserting desire or will, the ability to experience a range of emotions, initiating social contact, affection and warmth, social sensitivity, self-respect, acceptance of the needs of others, humour, creativity and self-expression, helpfulness and relaxation.[31] Dementia is a shared problem, for which adapting behaviours create a shared solution (Figure 3.2). A more inclusive and neurotolerant social infrastructure would enable richer lives for people with cognitive impairment.

## Mental health

Inequality and discrimination cause poor mental health just as they do poor physical health. Mental health diagnoses intersect with other conditions, increasing mortality and co-morbidity. Mental illness carries a huge cost, both societally and individually (Table 3.3), affecting one in four adults in

*Table 3.3* Mental illness

| | |
|---|---|
| Burden | Mental illness accounts for 32% of years lived with a disability.[a] |
| Prevalence of mental health conditions, adults, England[b] | 8% anxiety and depression<br>4% PTSD<br>3% depression<br>2% bipolar disorder<br>2–3% personality disorder<br><1% psychotic disorders |
| Prevalence of dementia | Around 900,000 people live with dementia in the UK, though only around 500,000 have a diagnosis.[c] |
| Children and young people, UK[d] | Rates of anxiety in young people have more than tripled in 15 years. Rates of depression, self harm, ASD and ADHD have doubled. |
| Mortality | Having schizophrenia more than triples one's risk of dying.[e] People in contact with mental health services have up to five times the death rates from some diseases.[f] People with severe mental illness die 15 to 20 years younger than the general population.[g] |
| Costs | By 2026, the annual cost of poor mental health in England is estimated to be £47 bn in service costs and £41 bn in lost earnings.[h] |

Notes:
a  Vigo D, Thornicroft G, Atun R. Estimating the true global burden of mental illness. *Lancet Psychiatry*. 2016;3(2):171–178. doi:10.1016/S2215-0366(15)00505-2.
b  *Mental Health and Wellbeing in England: Adult Psychiatric Morbidity Survey 2014*. NHS Digital;2014.https://digital.nhs.uk/data-and-information/publications/statistical/adult-psychiatric-morbidity-survey/adult-psychiatric-morbidity-survey-survey-of-mental-health-and-wellbeing-england-2014
c  Alzheimer's Society. *Dementia UK Prevalence Estimate for 2021: Methodology*.; 2021. https://www.alzheimers.org.uk/sites/default/files/2021-12/Dementia%20UK%20prevalence%20estimate%20for%202021%20methodology.pdf
d  Cybulski L, Ashcroft DM, Carr MJ, et al. Temporal trends in annual incidence rates for psychiatric disorders and self-harm among children and adolescents in the UK, 2003–2018. *BMC Psychiatry*. 2021;21(1):229. doi:10.1186/s12888-021-03235-w.
e  Olfson M, Gerhard T, Huang C, Crystal S, Stroup TS. Premature mortality among adults with schizophrenia in the United States. *JAMA Psychiatry*. 2015;72(12):1172. doi:10.1001/jamapsychiatry.2015.1737.
f  Public Health England. *Psychosis Data Report: Describing Variation in Numbers of People with Psychosis and Their Access to Care in England*. Public Health England; 2016:77. https://assets.publishing.service.gov.uk/government/uploads/system/uploads/attachment_data/file/774680/Psychosis_data_report.pdf
g  Public Health England. *Severe Mental Illness (SMI) and Physical Health Inequalities: Briefing*.; 2018. https://www.gov.uk/government/publications/severe-mental-illness-smi-physical-health-inequalities/severe-mental-illness-and-physical-health-inequalities-briefing
h  McCrone PR, ed. *Paying the Price: The Cost of Mental Health Care in England to 2026*. King's Fund; 2008. https://www.kingsfund.org.uk/sites/default/files/Paying-the-Price-the-cost-of-mental-health-care-England-2026-McCrone-Dhanasiri-Patel-Knapp-Lawton-Smith-Kings-Fund-May-2008_0.pdf

England in any one year. Awareness of mental health has increased in the last decade or so, along with rising rates of diagnosis, particularly in children and young people. While some of this is due to better recognition and reduced stigma, there are clear signs that our young people are struggling. The proportions of girls over twelve years old dissatisfied with their appearance doubled in the five years up to 2014.[32] Children living in more deprived areas are less likely to be referred for specialist help, even though they are more at risk. Much of the concern facing our young people is very real; anxiety is a rational response to climate and societal breakdown.

Defining what counts as mental health has become more blurred, with the term now used more often and in wider circumstances. Increasingly, there is a shift towards framing brief, normative stressful experiences such as anxiety before an exam in terms of being a mental health problem, which risks pathologising rather than promoting resilience. In clinical practice, there is no one point at which a patient's story starts becoming 'mental health'. Deciding to call something mental or physical health is rarely helpful, except when a referral is made, when navigating the complicated separation between the two cultures begins.

Poor mental health can manifest in many ways: psychosis, depression, anxiety, compulsions, somatisation, distress and trauma reactions, along with the psychological aspects of other chronic conditions. Major psychoses such as schizophrenia and bipolar disorder are considered severe and enduring mental illnesses (SMI), although these diseases affect more than the mind. There are widespread, consistent physical, metabolic and imaging changes demonstrable in people with SMI. Antipsychotic medications increase the risk of metabolic syndrome, the interaction between the vascular risk factors of raised sugar and cholesterol, high blood pressure and obesity.

Schizophrenia more than doubles the risk of dementia, even after adjusting for other risk factors,[33] and indeed was first described as precocious dementia, *dementia praecox* (Emil Kraepelin).[34] Although dementia has been considered part of the disease process of schizophrenia, damage may be due to medication rather than the condition. The argument that antipsychotic medication is neuroprotective has been used to justify longer term use of medication, but earlier withdrawal of medicines may prevent the long-term sequelae of chronic use of psychoactive medication.[35]

Schizophrenia is a disorder of the social brain, but it may have persisted as an evolutionary adaptation. The link with creativity could be the adaptive element which has continued to select for the expression of schizotypal traits.[36] New ideas tend to come from those on the edges of our societies.

## Diagnosis

Controlling the definitions of mental illness carries significant power. Psychiatry defines mental health disorders by consensus, on the grounds of expert opinion. There is no unity to mental health diagnoses, which are not dispassionate, objective representations, but instead culturally defined and curated by professionals (Michel Foucault). This view posits madness as a construct used to control those who think differently,[37] imposing the results of a medical hegemony on patients. Mental health services retain the right to impose treatment, a power that is open to misuse. Mental health care has the potential to be used as a tool to victimise and dehumanise diversity (Thomas Szasz).

Personality disorder is a problematic diagnostic realm, as the conclusion that symptoms are due to a disordered personality has a finality about it that blocks narratives of progress. Recognising the effects of adverse childhood experiences is a trauma-informed way to explain why some patterns of behaviour develop and persist into adulthood. It is far harder to build a stable life on unstable foundations. Patients diagnosed with borderline personality disorder are 13 times more likely to have experienced childhood adversity, in particular emotional abuse and neglect. Society scapegoats those who have been abused, rejecting the behaviours that result from maltreatment. A personality disorder diagnosis has too often been pejorative within mental health services, any challenge being attributed to and reinforcing the diagnosis. Those who resist are labelled non-compliant with medical authority.

Psychiatry has long been misused to reinforce establishment power. Mental health diagnoses were used to justify racism and oppression, by coining pseudo-conditions such as *drapetomania*, a supposed mental illness that makes a slave abscond.[38] Another supposed condition, *dysaesthesia Aethiopis*, caused 'rascality' in slaves who resisted the subservient role allocated them by the 'wisdom, mercy and justice' of the bible.

A century later, medicine was still supporting racism through the subjectivity of mental health diagnoses. Schizophrenia was considered a predominantly Black disease in the 1960s, with the label of *protest psychosis* used to devalue those active within the civil rights movement.[39] A hallmark of this diagnosis was 'denial of Caucasian values and hostility thereto'. Not treating or informing Black patients in the Tuskegee syphilis study (1932–1972) still influences trust in vaccination and enrolment in clinical trials by people of ethnic minority.[40]

Oppressive regimes such as the Soviet Union also found medicine a useful tool for dealing with dissidents. To complain about the political system under Stalin was clearly to be mad, which conveniently allowed the incarceration of those who threatened the regime. Punitive psychiatry cleared away any resistance while avoiding public scrutiny. Medicalisations of otherness are useful to authorities, helping focus discord on those outside the group, and by doing so claiming credit for raising the alarm. This is an important boundary which needs to be maintained and protected from misuse.

The dialogue around joblessness is an example of slippage towards state-controlled definitions of mental health. Proposals to put talking therapies workers into jobcentres endorse a neoliberal view that equates joblessness with deficit and disease. Mandatory courses designed to 'activate' those receiving welfare benefits impose interventions which aim to modify attitudes, pathologising difference and dissent.[41] Therapy coerced on the precariat in this way is unethical, as consent is not freely given when subsistence is tied to attendance. Using workfare sanctions to delegitimise labour does not lead to sustained increases in employment rates, but this is not the purpose; creating a transient workforce allows corporations to treat employees as disposable, obviating any need to improve working conditions.[42]

## Distress

A common factor underlying a decision to seek help is distress. Within Western medicine, this is most easily seen as a symptom of depression or anxiety, a way to simplify the complex of interacting factors that have led to this situation.[43] This dismisses sociosomatic causes and locates the problem as being one of individual weakness.

Distress is often a rational response to a dysfunctional situation, especially when lacking control over one's situation, which lowers one's sense of coherence. Distress manifests along the intersection of the interpersonal, social and political aspects of our lives, while *weltschmerz* ('world-pain') describes anguish at the state of the world, compared with how we think it should be. Pills are not a treatment for existential distress. Exploring narratives other than the biomedical opens up new ways to address the causes of distress.

The medicalisation of distress has seen antidepressant prescriptions rise both in absolute numbers (Figure 3.3) and as a share of overall prescriptions. Happiness scores have not changed (Figure 3.4). Antidepressants are vital

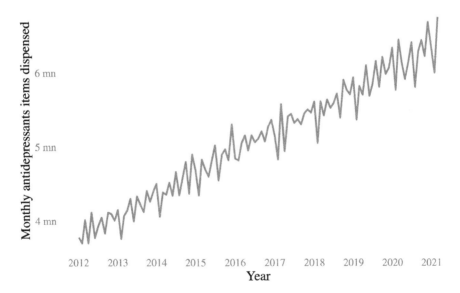

*Figure 3.3* Antidepressant prescriptions per month.

NHS Business Services Authority. Prescription Cost Analysis (PCA) data. Published online 2022. https://www.nhsbsa.nhs.uk/prescription-data/dispensing-data/prescription-cost-analysis-pca-data

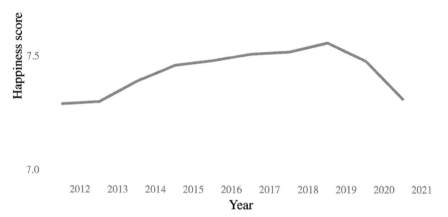

*Figure 3.4* Happiness scores over time, UK.

Office for National Statistics. Dataset: Annual personal well-being estimates. Published online October 15, 2021. https://www.ons.gov.uk/peoplepopulationandcommunity/wellbeing/bulletins/measuringnationalwellbeing/april2020tomarch2021/relateddata

medicines for many people, but approaches such as exercise, guided self-help and talking therapies such as CBT and behavioural activation are at least as cost-effective as medication for treating mild to moderate depression.[44]

The conventional explanation for the action of most antidepressants is that they raise serotonin levels within the brain, although there is actually little evidence for this.[45] All treatments for depression work by introducing perspective, a view from a different angle which helps find a way past a problem. The chain of negative thoughts feeding isolation can be broken anywhere; addressing isolation helps to address low mood. Spending time with others brings perspective, which opens up options. Increasing socialisation is effective mental health care.

Medical textbooks still describe mood disorders as primary (endogenous) or secondary to another cause (exogenous), although the treatment is the same. Comparing melancholia and mourning demonstrates the similarities between grieving and depression, in which one mourns the loss of an ideal as one would a person (Sigmund Freud).[46] The same process of loss and adjustment is occurring, but it is easier to understand the cause of distress when a loss is apparent. This brings more external support than the loss of a less visible, less tangible ideal.

Working through loss needs acceptance and forgiveness to resolve the anger, denial and guilt that accompanies grieving and bereavement (Elisabeth Kübler-Ross).[47] Change, and our resistance to accepting it, is a powerful source of distress. Healing comes from adapting to a new situation. The losses caused by life events, retirement and ill health all force change and adaptation, but our resilience to these varies. Association buffers this by increasing our sense of cohesion. Social capital and community support protect us as individuals, building our resilience to shocks. Outcomes are better in those who are more connected.

Healthcare has an important role to play in improving mental health, but in doing so has medicalised many aspects of normality. Short consultation times, patient pressure, long waiting lists or treatments being unavailable all drive practitioners towards prescribing medications. A majority of GPs would prescribe fewer antidepressants if other options were available to them.[48]

Good mental health is the most important factor in life satisfaction, more than physical aspects such as mobility.[49] Prevention has a vital role in improving mental health, but this happens outside of healthcare; a chat with a friend in a park or pub has powerful therapeutic and preventative value. Our ability to adapt and cope comes from our connections and the groups we are members of, our social capital protecting us.

## Symptomatology

Many symptoms do not have a diagnosable medical cause. Nearly half of all GP consultations do not lead to a diagnosis.[50] Much of what presents to doctors has no clinical explanation, and reassurance may be all that is needed for restitution. Many symptoms are normal physiological responses, but distress amplifies the experience of those symptoms, and their meaning. The degree of suffering experienced correlates poorly with the degree of injury or illness.[51] It is the significance and meaning of symptoms to the individual that lead to help seeking.

All chronic illness has a psychological component, including the shift of identity to becoming a 'patient' and the loss of power that entails. From the moment a decision has been made to seek help, the locus of control shifts. This is a measure of where power is located; an external locus comes from lacking belief in control over one's destiny, under the influence of others.[52] An internal locus lets us take arms against a sea of troubles.

The conflict between whether symptoms are physical rather than psychological dates back to Descartes.[53] Cartesian dualism separated mind and body, leading to an ongoing schism in medicine, within both our collective understanding and the structures of healthcare. Symptoms are simultaneously felt within the body and perceived by the mind, so any distinction between the two is necessarily arbitrary.

Health anxiety develops from concern about symptoms, worry causing physical sensations which become overwhelming, reinforcing a cycle of anxiety. A diagnosis that explains symptoms can be validating, especially for those with a large symptom burden. One catchall diagnosis calls these 'medically unexplained symptoms' (MUS), although the mechanisms are well understood. Symptoms are often triggered by acute illness, but the failure is in the restitution of health. Bodies remain in a state of high alertness, hyper-vigilance leading to unrefreshing sleep and the release of stress hormones. Upregulated nerve endings become hypersensitive, amplifying coenaesthetic awareness of physical symptoms. Anxiety exacerbates symptoms, reinforcing anxiety. Although somatisation often falls into culturally appropriate ways to articulate distress,[54] consultations can resemble symptom blizzards as distress spills over into the consulting room.

Symptoms that do not have a cultural or medical explanation are frustrating to patient and clinician alike. *Symptom shift* relocates difficult sensations as test results come back negative. Diseases that act like this are unusual but not inconceivable. A cycle of tests and referrals reduces clinical anxiety but can reinforce patient concern, leading to much low-value healthcare. A diagnosis of MUS medicalises symptoms while fending off any challenge to professional competency in the face of an unresolving condition.[55]

Considering these symptom clusters to be medically unexplored stories is a more productive way to explore this complex territory.[56] Discovering narratives helps to reach a shared understanding, creating a story that invites recovery.[57] There are elements of cognitive therapy in this approach, such as using reframing to provide an alternative view. Narrative based techniques take the view that a patient's story is broken, but locating the fault in a mutable object such as a story facilitates healing.

People in distress may seek help across multiple entry points, rejection sometimes intensifying attempts to access help. These patients become labelled as frequent attenders, a loaded term within healthcare. The vicar or faith leader, police, social worker and surgery are often dealing with the same individuals, each bringing their own institutional assumptions. The lack of shared record combined with rigid policies around consent and confidentiality make it hard to recognise or work jointly to meet needs.

The professionalisation of health-creation is just one facet of the commodification of our lives. Our health has been outsourced to institutions who relieve us of the responsibility for self-care, taking on the prevention and ownership of our wellbeing. 'Serviceland' takes over, as organisations identify deficits for their services to fix.[58] The powerlessness this creates becomes self-fulfilling, generating a passivity which induces a shift from citizen to consumer.

This power is not lost, but becomes transferred to institutions. Consultations inherit this power differential, driven by the asymmetric distribution of knowledge. The trappings of professional life, Latin words and the scattered arcana of medical devices reinforce authority. The imbalance of power drives *transference*, the unconscious projection of feelings onto another such as a care-giver. Consultation models such as transactional analysis highlight the similarities between the clinician-patient relationship and those of a parent and child. Transference and *countertransference* (the caregiver's reaction) also happen outside of traditional therapeutic relationships, for instance with volunteers, and it is helpful to recognise when this is happening. Peer support and supervision helps to identify and manage these situations.

### Does more healthcare make us more healthy?

Spending more on healthcare does not always lead to better health. Self reported health in particular gets worse with more healthcare. Comparing the United States with poor and rich areas of India shows that self-reported morbidity is highest in areas with the best health (as measured by life expectancy), while people in the poorest areas were far less likely to perceive themselves as being unwell.[59]

Medical care makes up only a small proportion of health outcomes. Health outcomes are affected mainly by social and economic factors, health behaviours and the environment, with only 20 per cent due to clinical care (Figure 3.5).[60] Funding does not match the distribution of causes. Healthcare spending may not be the most effective way to improve health; investing in social care achieves the same reduction in mortality at less than half the cost of healthcare or public health.[61]

Healthcare itself is not particularly good for our health. All medical investigations risk causing harm, from the test itself as well as the anxiety having a test brings. Overtreatment driven by fear of litigation is far more of a problem than undertreatment, though it is rare for people to complain about overtreatment. Doing something for the sake of being seen to do something, known as commission bias, drives a lot of unnecessary care. Shared understanding of the risks of medicalisation is important.

Costs and harms from healthcare increase with resources as activity increases, but the benefits are subject to the law of diminishing returns. There is a point of optimally effective care beyond which extra investment causes more harm than good (Figure 3.6).[62]

Of course, addressing the upstream determinants of disease would undermine the need for healthcare, which is a major contributor to economic activity; the UK spends one pound in every ten on healthcare. Corporate

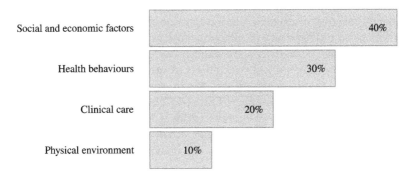

*Figure 3.5* Influence of factors on health outcomes.

County Health Rankings Scientific Advisory Group. *County Health Rankings and Roadmaps.* University of Wisconsin Population Health Institute; 2022. https://www.countyhealthrankings.org/explore-health-rankings/measures-data-sources/county-health-rankings-model

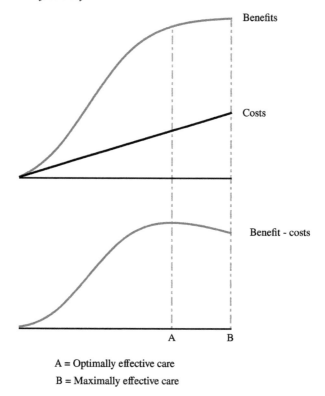

A = Optimally effective care
B = Maximally effective care

*Figure 3.6* Useful additions to care.

Muir Gray called this graph 'perhaps the most important picture in healthcare'. Donabedian A. *An Introduction to Quality Assurance in Health Care.* Oxford University Press; 2003.

prioritisation of shareholder value pulls more people into the expensive healthcare system. Paying providers by activity rewards quantity not quality, producing reactive, interventional, lower-value care.

Promising a pill for every ill, pharmaceutical companies are ever present within medicine. New drugs are eagerly welcomed into guidelines, the majority of which are subject to conflicts of interest.[63] Doctors accept that pharmaceutical sponsorship affects the prescribing habits of others but still believe themselves immune.[64] Direct-to-patient advertising stimulates demand, but another way to increase sales is to widen the potential pool of patients. Patient organisations that advocate for more identification and treatment of particular diseases are increasingly funded by the drug industry.[65]

Expanding diagnosis parameters opens up markets. Until 2009, child growth charts in the UK were based on formula fed infants,[66] who have faster weight gain than those who are breastfed. Setting normal values for weight as those of formula fed babies left some breastfed babies assessed as being underweight, pushing mothers to purchase formula and lose the benefits of breastfeeding.

Commercial influences have taken precedence over moral ones. Sharing techniques with the tobacco industry,[67] formula manufacturers put the needs of shareholders before those of babies by maximising sales,[68] despite the harms from reducing or stopping breastfeeding. Giving free samples of formula milk creates dependent customers, as maternal milk production stops when not feeding. Universal breastfeeding would prevent over 800,000 deaths of preschool children and 20,000 deaths from breast cancer each year.[69]

Targets for treatment have become more aggressive over time. Loosening of criteria for diagnosis casts the net of disease yet wider. Risk factors are converted into diseases such as pre-diabetes, a rise in blood sugar that represents a risk but not at a level that diagnoses diabetes. As thresholds get lowered and these pre-diseases become normalised, modern medicine becomes an industry, generating illness rather than health. Ivan Illich describes this as *social iatrogenesis*,[70] medical hegemony reinforcing a morbid society. Illich suggests that institutions become more likely to cause harm as they grow.[71] Incorporating the economics of scarcity reinforces healthcare as the main producer of health, which disenfranchises individuals and communities from taking control.

### Salutogenesis and wellbeing

Rather than looking for deficits that need mending, we could instead support things that are good for our health. *Salutogenesis* recognises those factors which are health-creating (Aaron Antonovsky).[72] Identifying assets rather than deficiencies shifts our view to an alternative with more possibilities. Inverting concepts of illness, *wellbeing* describes our satisfaction with our lives, reflecting our sense of control and purpose, how we function and how happy we feel. While our sense of wellbeing is subjective, our circumstances such as work, education and housing give some level of objective measure.

Wellbeing comparisons include both an individual's subjective experience of life and an objective comparison of life and social circumstances.[73] Wellbeing and health outcomes are closely correlated. Improving wellbeing benefits health, particularly immune functioning and protection from stress.[74]

Wellbeing can be measured at individual, community and national level. Individually, the Warwick-Edinburgh Mental Wellbeing Scale (WEMWBS)[75] is a validated seven- or fourteen- item questionnaire measuring wellbeing and psychological functioning. This takes a more holistic approach, with questions about optimism, confidence and feeling loved having relevance to real lives. Measuring wellbeing scores regularly over a period of time helps to show which aspects of our lives make the most difference to our wellbeing.

*Table 3.4* Measures of national wellbeing (ONS)[a]

| | |
|---|---|
| Personal wellbeing | Satisfaction with life, worthiness of what we do, anxiety, happiness |
| Relationships | Loneliness, people to rely on, happiness of relationships |
| Health | Healthy life expectancy at birth, disability, satisfaction with health, depression or anxiety |
| Activities | Employment, job satisfaction, leisure time satisfaction, volunteering, participation in culture and in sports |
| Housing | Crime, feeling safe, access to natural environment, neighbourliness, access to key services, satisfaction with accommodation |
| Personal finance | Low income, wealth, income and satisfaction with income, financial difficulties |
| Economy | Disposable income, public sector debt, inflation |
| Education | Human capital, qualifications, numbers who are NEET (not in education, employment or training) |
| Governance | Voter turnout, trust in government |
| Environment | Greenhouse gas emissions, protected areas, renewable energy, recycling |

Note:
a  Office for National Statistics. *Measures of National Well-Being Dashboard*. ONS; 2019. https://www.ons.gov.uk/peoplepopulationandcommunity/wellbeing/articles/measuresofnationalwellbeingdashboard/2018-09-26

Humans have always debated how to maximise human happiness and wellbeing. Aristotle used the term *eudaimonia*, which literally means having a good demon, as distinguished from hedonic enjoyment, seeking pleasure. The idea of virtue was central to such flourishing, with friendship a key virtue in achieving this positive state. Eudaimonia is best understood as the type of life that can be looked back on and say 'it was well lived'. Friendship, and purpose, allows us to achieve this.

*Five ways to wellbeing* condenses millennia of advice on how to live well and stay healthy into five principles[76]:

- **connect** with people
- stay **active**
- take **notice**, staying aware of the present moment
- continue to **learn**
- **give** time or skills

These provide an excellent framework for evidence-based approaches to wellbeing. The benefits of social participation and connections to good mental health are well recognised, as are the interactions between physical activity and subjective wellbeing. Mindful approaches encourage choices in keeping with personal values, moving the locus of control closer,[77] which helps to sustain positive behavioural changes. Continuing to learn as an adult improves self-esteem and increases opportunities for social interactions, demonstrating how each of the five ways reinforces the others. The search for meaning is a universal human need. Participation in community life brings meaning and satisfaction, as volunteers know. This is where the health benefits of community are realised.

## Notes

Links and additional resources for this chapter can be found at www.communityhealth. uk/3-disorders-of-society

1 Berkman L, Syme SL. Social networks, host resistance and mortality: a nine-year follow-up study of Alameda County residents. *Am J Epidemiol.* 1979;109(2):186–204. doi:10.1093/oxfordjournals.aje.a112674.

2 Cacioppo JT, Hawkley LC, Ernst JM, et al. Loneliness within a nomological net: an evolutionary perspective. *J Res Personal.* 2006;40(6):1054–1085. doi:10.1016/j.jrp.2005.11.007.

3 Qualter P, Vanhalst J, Harris R, et al. Loneliness across the life span. *Perspect Psychol Sci.* 2015;10(2):250–264. doi:10.1177/1745691615568999.

4 Jopling, Kate. *Combatting Loneliness One Conversation at a Time.* Jo Cox Commission on Loneliness; 2017. https://www.jocoxfoundation.org/loneliness_commission

5 Office for National Statistics. *Loneliness - What Characteristics and Circumstances Are Associated with Feeling Lonely?* ONS; 2018. https://www.ons.gov.uk/peoplepopulationandcommunity/wellbeing/articles/lonelinesswhatcharacteristicsandcircumstancesareassociatedwithfeelinglonely/2018-04-10

6 Harris RA, Qualter P, Robinson SJ. Loneliness trajectories from middle childhood to pre-adolescence: impact on perceived health and sleep disturbance. *J Adolesc.* 2013;36(6):1295–1304. doi:10.1016/j.adolescence.2012.12.009.

7 Qualter, Pamela. *Tackling Loneliness Evidence Review: Main Report.* Dept for Digital, Culture, Media and Sport, UK Government; 2022. https://www.gov.uk/government/publications/tackling-loneliness-evidence-review/tackling-loneliness-evidence-review-full-report

8 Caspi A, Harrington H, Moffitt TE, Milne BJ, Poulton R. Socially isolated children 20 years later: risk of cardiovascular disease. *Arch Pediatr Adolesc Med.* 2006;160(8):805. doi:10.1001/archpedi.160.8.805.

9 Nyqvist F, Victor CR, Forsman AK, Cattan M. The association between social capital and loneliness in different age groups: a population-based study in Western Finland. *BMC Public Health.* 2016;16(1):542. doi:10.1186/s12889-016-3248-x.

10 See note 5.

11 Department for Digital, Culture, Media and Sport. *A Connected Society: A Strategy for Tackling Loneliness – Laying the Foundations for Change.* UK Government; 2018. https://www.gov.uk/guidance/governments-work-on-tackling-loneliness

12 Barreto M, Victor C, Hammond C, Eccles A, Richins MT, Qualter P. Loneliness around the world: age, gender, and cultural differences in loneliness. *Personal Individ Differ.* 2021;169:110066. doi:10.1016/j.paid.2020.110066.

13 Christiansen J, Qualter P, Friis K, et al. Associations of loneliness and social isolation with physical and mental health among adolescents and young adults. *Perspect Public Health.* 2021;141(4):226–236. doi:10.1177/17579139211016077.

14 Herlitz J, Wiklund I, Caidahl K, et al. The feeling of loneliness prior to coronary artery bypass grafting might be a predictor of short- and long-term postoperative mortality. *Eur J Vasc Endovasc Surg.* 1998;16(2):120–125. doi:10.1016/S1078-5884(98)80152-4.

15 Gove WR. Sex, marital status, and mortality. *Am J Sociol.* 1973;79(1):45–67. doi:10.1086/225505.

16 Cohen S. Psychosocial vulnerabilities to upper respiratory infectious illness: implications for susceptibility to coronavirus disease 2019 (COVID-19). *Perspect Psychol Sci.* 2021;16(1):161–174. doi:10.1177/1745691620942516.

17 Cacioppo JT, Hawkley LC, Berntson GG, et al. Do lonely days invade the nights? Potential social modulation of sleep efficiency. *Psychol Sci.* 2002;13(4):384–387. doi:10.1111/1467-9280.00469.

18 Holt-Lunstad J, Smith TB, Layton JB. Social relationships and mortality risk: a meta-analytic review. Brayne C, ed. *PLoS Med.* 2010;7(7):e1000316. doi:10.1371/journal.pmed.1000316.

19 Putnam RD. *Bowling Alone: The Collapse and Revival of American Community.* Simon & Schuster; 2001.

20 Routasalo PE, Tilvis RS, Kautiainen H, Pitkala KH. Effects of psychosocial group rehabilitation on social functioning, loneliness and well-being of lonely, older people: randomized controlled trial. *J Adv Nurs.* 2009;65(2):297–305. doi:10.1111/j.1365-2648.2008.04837.x.

21 Eccles AM, Qualter P. Review: Alleviating loneliness in young people – a meta-analysis of interventions. *Child Adolesc Ment Health.* 2021;26(1):17–33. doi:10.1111/camh.12389.

22 Ibarra F, Baez M, Cernuzzi L, Casati F. A systematic review on technology-supported interventions to improve old-age social wellbeing: loneliness, social isolation, and connectedness. *J Healthc Eng.* 2020;2020:1–14. doi:10.1155/2020/2036842.

23 McDaid, David, Park, A-La, Fernandez, Jose-Luis. *Reconnections: Impact Evaluation, Final Report.* London Schools of Economics and Political Science; 2021:43. https://www.lse.ac.uk/cpec/assets/documents/Reconnections.pdf

24 Masi CM, Chen HY, Hawkley LC, Cacioppo JT. A meta-analysis of interventions to reduce loneliness. *Personal Soc Psychol Rev.* 2011;15(3):219–266. doi:10.1177/1088868310377394.

25 Alzheimer's Research UK. Dementia diagnoses in the UK. Dementia Statistics Hub. https://www.dementiastatistics.org/statistics/diagnoses-in-the-uk/

26 Wilson RS, Krueger KR, Arnold SE, et al. Loneliness and risk of Alzheimer disease. *Arch Gen Psychiatry.* 2007;64(2):234. doi:10.1001/archpsyc.64.2.234.

27 Boss L, Kang DH, Branson S. Loneliness and cognitive function in the older adult: a systematic review. *Int Psychogeriatr.* 2015;27(4):541–553. doi:10.1017/S1041610214002749.

28 Donovan NJ, Okereke OI, Vannini P, et al. Association of Higher Cortical Amyloid Burden With Loneliness in Cognitively Normal Older Adults. *JAMA Psychiatry.* 2016;73(12):1230. doi:10.1001/jamapsychiatry.2016.2657.

29 Sundström A, Adolfsson AN, Nordin M, Adolfsson R. Loneliness increases the risk of all-cause dementia and Alzheimer's Disease. Anderson N, ed. *J Gerontol Ser B.* 2020;75(5):919–926. doi:10.1093/geronb/gbz139.

30 Kitwood T, Bredin K. Towards a theory of dementia care: personhood and well-being. *Ageing Soc.* 1992;12(03):269–287. doi:10.1017/S0144686X0000502X.

31 Ibid.

32 Morgan C, Webb RT, Carr MJ, et al. Incidence, clinical management, and mortality risk following self harm among children and adolescents: cohort study in primary care. *BMJ.* Published online October 18, 2017:j4351. doi:10.1136/bmj.j4351.

33 Fischer CE, Agüera-Ortiz L. Psychosis and dementia: risk factor, prodrome, or cause? *Int Psychogeriatr.* 2018;30(2):209–219. doi:10.1017/S1041610217000874.

34 Adityanjee, Aderibigbe YA, Theodoridis D, Vieweg WVR. Dementia praecox to schizophrenia: The first 100 years. *Psychiatry Clin Neurosci.* 1999;53(4):437–448. doi:10.1046/j.1440-1819.1999.00584.x.

35 Moncrieff J. Questioning the 'neuroprotective' hypothesis: does drug treatment prevent brain damage in early psychosis or schizophrenia? *Br J Psychiatry.* 2011;198(2):85–87. doi:10.1192/bjp.bp.110.085795.

36 Burns JK. An evolutionary theory of schizophrenia: Cortical connectivity, metarepresentation, and the social brain. *Behav Brain Sci.* 2004;27(6):831–855. doi:10.1017/S0140525X04000196.
37 Middleton H, Shaw I. Inequalities in mental health: Models and explanations. *Policy Polit.* 1999;27(1):43–55. doi:10.1332/030557399782019499.
38 Cartwright, Samuel. Report on the diseases and physical peculiarities of the Negro race. *New Orleans Med Surg J.* May 1851:707–715.
39 Bromberg W. The 'protest' psychosis: a special type of reactive psychosis. *Arch Gen Psychiatry.* 1968;19(2):155. doi:10.1001/archpsyc.1968.01740080027005.
40 Corbie-Smith G. The continuing legacy of the Tuskegee syphilis study: considerations for clinical investigation: *Am J Med Sci.* 1999;317(1):5–8. doi:10.1097/00000441-199901000-00002.
41 Friedli L, Stearn R. Positive affect as coercive strategy: conditionality, activation and the role of psychology in UK government workfare programmes. *Med Humanit.* 2015;41(1):40–47. doi:10.1136/medhum-2014-010622.
42 Briken K, Taylor P. Fulfilling the 'British way': beyond constrained choice – Amazon workers' lived experiences of workfare. *Ind Relat J.* 2018;49(5–6):438–458. doi:10.1111/irj.12232.
43 Dowrick C. *Beyond Depression: A New Approach to Understanding and Management.* Oxford University Press; 2004.
44 NICE guideline. *Depression in Adults: Treatment and Management.* National Institute for Health and Care Excellence; 2022. https://www.nice.org.uk/guidance/ng222
45 Moncrieff J, Cooper RE, Stockmann T, Amendola S, Hengartner MP, Horowitz MA. The serotonin theory of depression: a systematic umbrella review of the evidence. *Mol Psychiatry.* Published online July 20, 2022. doi:10.1038/s41380-022-01661-0.
46 Freud, Sigmund. Mourning and melancholia. *Stand Ed.* 1917;14(239):1957–1961.
47 Kübler-Ross E. *On Death and Dying.* Tavistock / Routledge; 1989.
48 Halliwell E. *Up and Running? Exercise Therapy and the Treatment of Mild or Moderate Depression in Primary Care.* Mental Health Foundation; 2005. https://www.bl.uk/collection-items/up-and-running-exercise-therapy-and-the-treatment-of-mild-or-moderate-depression-in-primary-care
49 Layard, Richard, Clark, David M. *Annexes to THRIVE: The Revolutionary Potential of Evidence-Based Psychological Therapies.* London School of Economics and Political Science; 2013. https://cep.lse.ac.uk/layard/thriveannex.pdf
50 Thomas KB. Temporarily dependent patient in general practice. *BMJ.* 1974;1(5908):625–626. doi:10.1136/bmj.1.5908.625.
51 Fields HL. Pain modulation: expectation, opioid analgesia and virtual pain. In: *Progress in Brain Research.* Vol 122. Elsevier; 2000:245–253. doi:10.1016/S0079-6123(08)62143-3.
52 Rotter JB. Generalized expectancies for internal versus external control of reinforcement. *Psychol Monogr Gen Appl.* 1966;80(1):1–28. doi:10.1037/h0092976.
53 Fitzpatrick M. Myalgic encephalomyelitis--the dangers of Cartesian fundamentalism. *Br J Gen Pract J R Coll Gen Pract.* 2002;52(478):432–433.
54 Kleinman A, Becker AE. 'Sociosomatics': the contributions of anthropology to psychosomatic medicine. *Psychosom Med.* 1998;60(4):389–393. doi:10.1097/00006842-199807000-00001.
55 Kirmayer LJ, Groleau D, Looper KJ, Dao MD. Explaining medically unexplained symptoms. *Can J Psychiatry.* 2004;49(10):663–672. doi:10.1177/070674370404901003.
56 Launer J. Medically unexplored stories. *Postgrad Med J.* 2009;85(1007):503–504. doi:10.1136/pgmj.2009.087411.

57  Howard Brody. 'My story is broken; can you help me fix it?': Medical ethics and the joint construction of narrative. *Lit Med.* 1994;13(1):79–92. doi:10.1353/lm.2011.0169.

58  Russell C. *Rekindling Democracy: A Professional's Guide to Working in Citizen Space.* Cascade Books; 2020.

59  Sen A. Health: perception versus observation: Self reported morbidity has severe limitations and can be extremely misleading. *BMJ.* 2002;324(7342):860–861. doi:10.1136/bmj.324.7342.860.

60  County Health Rankings Scientific Advisory Group. *County Health Rankings and Roadmaps.* University of Wisconsin Population Health Institute; 2022. https://www.countyhealthrankings.org/explore-health-rankings/measures-data-sources/county-health-rankings-model

61  Martin S, Longo F, Lomas J, Claxton K. Causal impact of social care, public health and healthcare expenditure on mortality in England: cross-sectional evidence for 2013/2014. *BMJ Open.* 2021;11(10):e046417. doi:10.1136/bmjopen-2020-046417.

62  Gray M, Gray J, Howick J. Personalised healthcare and population healthcare. *J R Soc Med.* 2018;111(2):51–56. doi:10.1177/0141076817732523.

63  Norris SL, Holmer HK, Ogden LA, Burda BU. Conflict of interest in clinical practice guideline development: a systematic review. Mintzes B, ed. *PLoS ONE.* 2011;6(10):e25153. doi:10.1371/journal.pone.0025153.

64  Steinman MA, Shlipak MG, McPhee SJ. Of principles and pens: attitudes and practices of medicine housestaff toward pharmaceutical industry promotions. *Am J Med.* 2001;110(7):551–557. doi:10.1016/s0002-9343(01)00660-x.

65  Ozieranski P, Rickard E, Mulinari, S. Exposing drug industry funding of UK patient organisations. *BMJ.* Published online May 22, 2019:l1806. doi:10.1136/bmj.l1806.

66  Coombes R. UK adopts growth charts based on data from breastfed babies. *BMJ.* 2009;338:b1892. doi:10.1136/bmj.b1892.

67  Granheim Ionata S, Engelhardt K, Rundall P, Bialous S, Iellamo A, Margetts B. Interference in public health policy. *World Nutr.* 2017;8(2):288. doi:10.26596/wn.201782288-310.

68  Becker GE, Ching C, Nguyen TT, Cashin J, Zambrano P, Mathisen R. Babies before business: protecting the integrity of health professionals from institutional conflict of interest. *BMJ Glob Health.* 2022;7(8):e009640. doi:10.1136/bmjgh-2022-009640.

69  Victora CG, Bahl R, Barros AJD, et al. Breastfeeding in the 21st century: epidemiology, mechanisms, and lifelong effect. *The Lancet.* 2016;387(10017):475–490. doi:10.1016/S0140-6736(15)01024-7.

70  Illich I. *Medical Nemesis: The Expropriation of Health.* Calder & Boyars; 1974.

71  Russell C. Does more medicine make us sicker? Ivan Illich revisited. *Gac Sanit.* 2019;33(6):579–583. doi:10.1016/j.gaceta.2018.11.006.

72  Antonovsky A. The salutogenic model as a theory to guide health promotion. *Health Promot Int.* 1996;11(1):11–18. doi:10.1093/heapro/11.1.11.

73  World Health Organization. *Measurement of and Target-Setting for Well-Being: An Initiative by the WHO Regional Office for Europe.* Regional Office for Europe; 2013. https://apps.who.int/iris/handle/10665/107309

74  Howell RT, Kern ML, Lyubomirsky S. Health benefits: Meta-analytically determining the impact of well-being on objective health outcomes. *Health Psychol Rev.* 2007;1(1):83–136. doi:10.1080/17437190701492486.

75  Tennant R, Hiller L, Fishwick R, et al. The Warwick-Edinburgh Mental Wellbeing Scale (WEMWBS): development and UK validation. *Health Qual Life Outcomes.* 2007;5(1):63. doi:10.1186/1477-7525-5-63.

76  Aked, Jody, Marks, Nic, Cordon, Corrina, Thompson, Sam. *Five Ways to Wellbeing.* New Economics Foundation; 2008. https://neweconomics.org/2008/10/five-ways-to-wellbeing

77  Krasner M. Mindfulness-based interventions: a coming of age? *Fam Syst Health.* 2004;22(2):207–212. doi:10.1037/1091-7527.22.2.207.

# 4 Healthcare structures

The labyrinthine structures of healthcare are hard to navigate even for those working within the system. Services to address the health needs of the population have evolved in a reactive rather than a strategic way. Structural issues and perverse incentives have encouraged the generation of healthcare rather than health as the primary outcome. The complexity of healthcare systems can make them appear impenetrable to those looking to build bridges with health services.

Publicly funded healthcare in the UK is provided by the NHS, while social care, public health and prevention fall under local authority control, an arbitrary budgetary divide which has done much to frustrate joint working. These statutory services are directly commissioned by government to address the needs of the population. Alternative provision is by for-profit organisations and the 'third sector', which comprises the Voluntary and Community Sector (VCS), also known as Voluntary, Community and Social Enterprise (VCSE). This includes voluntary organisations, social enterprises, charities and public service mutuals, organisations hived off from the public sector. The difference between the sectors is based on funding streams: public, business and charity respectively, with third sector philanthropic funding the most precarious. Public funds are limited and remain vulnerable to political decisions, while privately funded services are at risk from extraction of value to shareholders.

Population-based care including health education, prevention and immunisation is the traditional responsibility of public health. Receiving just 4 per cent of NHS funding,[1] prevention remains the poor relative to the NHS, which spends many times this on primary care, and far more still on hospital-based care.[2] Public health budgets sit outside the usual NHS structures, funded instead by and answerable to local authorities. Local council oversight means public health departments are potentially more accountable to citizens than other healthcare providers. Splitting individual and population level healthcare thwarts projects that work across both levels.

DOI: 10.4324/9781003391784-5

## Prevention or cure?

There is an ongoing tension in healthcare funding between prevention and cure. Although it is almost always cheaper to prevent something than it is to fix it later, current funding favours reactive over proactive care. Healthcare jobs aim to make people better, not to stop them needing healthcare.[3] The need for better efforts at prevention is unarguable, but services are too busy intervening to look upstream at why people are becoming unwell. Decision-makers recognise the need for and cost-effectiveness of prevention, but resources tend not to follow the rhetoric. Innovation in reactive care dominates ideas about treatment and how money should be spent. The influence of the biomedical and pharmaceutical industries has led to incredible advances in healthcare, but steered by the need to maximise shareholder value rather than improve health.

A top-heavy view of health is reinforced by media portrayals of healthcare depicting hospitals and ambulances as a convenient journalistic shorthand for healthcare. The political expediency of maintaining hospitals as the most visible proxy for healthcare provision means that less glamorous approaches are often ignored by the media and the public. Successful prevention goes unnoticed and uncounted, but is the most effective healthcare: when a smoker stops, and doesn't get lung disease as a result. Reactive care instead promises redemption, that we can do the wrong thing and still get away with it. These indulgences let us continue to consume and ask forgiveness later.

Funding health interventions solely through healthcare providers professionalises responses and misses the ability of other departments to improve health outcomes. A 'health in all policies' approach recognises health-creating aspects throughout services, but needs joined-up working to ensure that approaches are consistent and congruent. This helps to avoid the inter-organisational holes into which fall issues that cross multiple departments but are funded by none.

If reactive care is the visible side of health, social care is the invisible side. The boundary between health and social care is fluid and arbitrary, leading to territorial squabbling over budgets. Preventative health meanwhile is left in the no-man's-land between different budgets, stressed organisations on each side of the funding gap reluctant to cede part of their budgets away from their own core priorities.

## Specialist care

The lion's share of healthcare funding goes to specialist, hospital-based care, which is by nature more expensive. Hospitals are a bad place to be ill, except for a selected group of patients for whom the benefits of intensive input outweigh the significant nosocomial harms of hospitalisation. Patients lose muscle strength with each day spent in bed, while limited visiting from loved ones and ward cultures that tidy patients back into their beds contribute to isolation, deconditioning and loss of independence.

Considering how few people want to be in hospital, they are surprisingly busy places. Loneliness and anxiety influence help-seeking. Being around other people is comforting, and the Emergency Department or GP surgery can be a reassuring and interesting place to be. Acute health services are based around the needs of symptomatic people, so making access to help dependent on production of symptoms leads to a focus on these.

Hospitals cannot be below a certain size, as all the various specialties depend on each other to work, just as the body's organs do. Hospital care carries the expectation of scans and admissions, but the same symptoms can often be managed with less arousal by other services. For patients with more complex symptomatology, the anxiety that investigations inevitably bring can hinder progress. Emergency departments are not set up to provide chronic disease care, but the erosion of other services has left work overflowing onto these more expensive acute services.

Community hospitals are a valuable asset, providing in- and out-patient care nearer to home. These health campuses can be an integral part of the community by inviting in the help of their wider patient group. Volunteer-supported activities bring the outside world in. These extra hands help with reablement, such as using games to build muscle strength and mobility.

## Care closer to home

The opposite of these large organisations is the traditional model of NHS primary care, independent practices run by GP partnerships providing services according to need. These clinically-led smaller organisations have endured by being flexible and adaptable. Everyone has access to a GP practice and an expectation of the service provided. Primary care takes all comers, managing acute problems, chronic disease, prevention and risk factor management.

There is a risk that using the terms primary and secondary care trap us into existing ways of thinking about care provision, which discourages innovation.[4] It is generalist and specialist healthcare that are being provided. Specialist clinics in the community usually follow a traditional outpatient model, but being based in GP practices and community buildings does not make these services primary care, which is a way of working, not the building a clinician works from. Primary care means direct access to appointments, guided by care navigation where needed. Shared records allow better continuity and less duplication of investigations. Trust in the assessments of colleagues is efficient and avoids the frustration of telling a story repeatedly.

General practice has survived by being nimble, with enough generic skills within teams to be able to cover across roles when needed, functioning as a 'universal sink plug' for the various holes in the system. That practices are independent businesses supports clinical autonomy and diversity, which helps resilience across the system. GP practices form a community asset channelling local social capital. Resourcing primary care is cost-effective, needing three times as many hospital doctors as GPs to achieve a similar improvement in mortality.[5] Outcomes are better with higher ratios of primary care physicians to population, improving life expectancy and mortality.[6]

Almost half the workload in primary care comes from a tenth of patients. This follows the rule that half of any workload is attributable to the square root of the number of people involved (Price's square root law). The most frequent attenders are usually episodic, with spells of high attendance due to acute illness, needing regular blood tests and reviews. This group typically represents fewer than 1 per cent of patients who are being closely managed through an acute illness or flare of chronic disease. The next group are more disparate, comprising approximately one in fifty patients who sees a GP more than monthly. A typical GP list of two thousand patients will have forty or so patients attending this often.

The factors underpinning a decision to seek help are many and complex. Previous experience of health care, stories of late or misdiagnosis and access to care all influence presentation. Hypervigilance and health anxiety are common. Seeking reassurance is often provoked by illness in someone close, when symptoms take on far more significance. Other issues such as lack of housing or access to benefits are also common contributors to presentations.

Healthcare services may inadvertently reinforce demand by inducing mutual dependency. A qualitative study of the consultations of a frequently attending family showed doctor and patient trapped in a dysfunctional relationship, as GP changes in their surgery influenced attendances.[7] Meanwhile, 30 per cent of patients do not see their GP in any one year. Most of these will not have any symptoms they consider worthy of attention or the effort of seeking help, but there are also those who actively avoid engagement with health services. These people may attract the label 'hard-to-reach', but we could instead consider what would make services more accessible while respecting the autonomy behind these decisions.

Patient pathways, as mapped out in commissioning meetings, finish with arrows pointing towards 'the community'. While on these journeys, patients are removed from their community by inference and sometimes in actuality. That reintegration into community might be considered to be needed at the end of an episode of care reflects the extent to which pathways have been medicalised. At worst, signposts all pointing away from healthcare reflect a colonial view of community services, surrounding and protecting the health citadel at all costs. 'Discharge to the community' often means a list of resources to be given to a patient, along with a letter explaining how they no longer need the team's help. Hands are washed.

The feeling of rejection that careless discharge brings can create a feeling of abandonment and despair, sometimes awakening trauma from previous losses, symptoms worsening as discharge approaches. High walls around specialist services created by referral thresholds and discharge criteria are used as a way of managing caseloads, but reinforce the separation of services and maintain difficulties in accessing help. Services avoid these issues by offering ongoing access without the need to be gatekept.

Being trapped within the wrong part of the system is also harmful, as well as expensive. Teams sometimes hold on tightly to their clients, even when not set up to deliver appropriate help. Recognising when other services are better placed for involvement is key to avoiding mutual dependency. A smoother transfer to more community-based input provides ongoing stepped-down, demedicalised support. Effective transfer of care requires identifying who is best placed to pick up ongoing need.

Breaking down these blocks between parts of the system allows patients to access appropriate help directly. In healthcare terms, providing navigational support to access the correct services is an effective way to demedicalise care and reduce the waste from duplication of effort.

## NHS structures

The organisational structures of healthcare in the UK are complex and ever-shifting, the only constant in the NHS being continual change. Despite the promise by the incoming coalition government in 2010 of no top-down NHS reorganisation, the 2012 Health and Social Care Act did exactly that. Clinical input into Primary Care Trusts (PCTs) had been via a professional executive, but the new change was promoted as putting clinicians at the heart of decision-making, replacing PCTs with Clinical Commissioning Groups (CCGs). This massive reshuffle left attention focused on structure rather than delivery, although it did encourage the involvement of clinical leaders in decisions and implement a legal duty to address health inequalities.

The change to clinical commissioning has made little difference to population outcomes. The restructuring of both CCGs and PCTs has failed to make a significant impact on health inequalities.[8] In particular, attempts to address inequalities due to ethnicity have remained peripheral, focused more on complying with legal requirements rather than being integral to policy.[9]

Each reorganisation changes the signage and stationery but hides an erosion of services. Politicians love to show mastery of the NHS by leaving their own mark, and while redesigns may not be part of any wider long-term strategy or have any value in healthcare terms, they generate media attention and the illusion of control and progress. Freeing the NHS from political micromanagement would encourage a longer-term approach to healthcare.[10]

Successive governments have tried to advance competition within healthcare, a triumph of free-market dogma over the lack of evidence that this is an effective way to arrange services. The idea behind the purchaser-provider split was to encourage other providers into healthcare, which would in turn drive up quality. In practice, the need for competitive procurement left commissioners cautious about developing new partnerships, leaving the playing field tilted towards large organisations with sufficient resources to engage with the bidding process. Introducing mechanisms by which private organisations can provide care on behalf of the NHS has allowed providers to cherry-pick profitable activity, leaving the NHS to deal with complex and more risky cases without the training opportunities and funding that more routine work brings.[11]

**Integrated care systems**

In an attempt to solve the boundary issues of cross-organisational working, providers and commissioners have been brought together to work from a shared budget in the form of integrated care systems (ICSs). There are forty-two ICSs in England, combining the functions of CCGs to work across larger areas. CCG footprints survive within this as 'place', a recognition that natural geographies may not fit organisational structures. ICSs are managed by integrated care boards (ICBs), statutory NHS organisations responsible for meeting the health needs of the population. Health boards and trusts fulfil a similar function in Scotland and Wales.

'Integrated' is one of the most overused terms in healthcare provision, usually implying a focus on system structures rather than the care being provided. Connecting parts of the system into something more whole is a fine ambition, but all should have a voice. Smaller providers such as GP practices are not resourced to be able to represent themselves within ICSs, shifting the playing field to benefit larger organisations. Federations representing GP practices let these small fish swim together as a shoal.

The economies of scale make smaller practices less viable, leading to GP practices being slowly subsumed into larger organisations. This brings some resilience but threatens the strength of traditional models of independent general practice. ICS structures may accelerate a shift from patient to consumer by opening up possibilities for competition, together with a policy to extend hours, which values convenience over continuity. The patients who make up the majority of primary care work would rather wait to see someone they know and trust.[12]

The aspiration for ICSs is to work more closely with communities through integrated care partnerships (ICPs), for example managing long-term conditions. This may be challenging to organisational cultures which have been encouraged to thrive by expanding rather than ceding territory.

**Primary care networks**

While commissioning functions have moved to larger ICSs, primary care networks (PCNs) now organise care delivery over a smaller footprint. The optimum size of these local health organisations is considered to be between 30,000 and 50,000 patients. This is big enough to justify more specialist staff working across practices, while being small enough to know each other. PCNs were formalised in 2019, requiring GP practices to collaborate with local colleagues to work at scale. Clinical time, management and a support team are funded, with payments to support the time for practices to engage. PCNs have moved us nearer to the idea of community being the smallest unit of health.[13]

The arrival of COVID-19 put these nascent networks centre stage and helped to forge relationships between practices, who worked together to cover urgent care and vaccination centres. With a shortage of trained GPs to do the work, the additional roles reimbursement scheme (ARRS) funds other health professionals to take on some primary care activity, the equivalent of vouchers rather than cash to direct spending. Additional roles include first contact practitioners (FCPs, musculoskeletal therapists), clinical pharmacists, health and wellbeing coaches and social prescribers, while ANPs (advanced nurse practitioners) and paramedics now see a large proportion of acute illness presentations. There has not been a corresponding expansion of training in these roles, so a lack of suitably skilled staff in these multidisciplinary roles is holding back a useful diversification of responses.

## Patient involvement

While many NHS documents boast of coproduction, true patient involvement remains rare. The intricacies of funding, contracting and service provision make informed decisions hard for patient groups. Commissioners translate central diktat into financial targets for providers to chase, while users of services have remarkably little say in the process. Lay people have only tokenistic representation into the way services are provided, patient involvement at the lowest level being to endorse decisions made by professionals on behalf of patients. When done well, this can provide helpful sense checking, but this still involves services being provided for, rather than with or by citizens. Patient views are rarely considered when defining problems to be solved, but improving public involvement in research allows patient-led priorities to influence the process of generating healthcare evidence.[14]

The most local layer of patient involvement is the Patient Participation Group (PPG). All GP surgeries should have a PPG that is reasonably representative of the practice population, to provide overview and patient feedback. PPGs open up opportunities for community involvement such as help with immunisation clinics, and can play an important role identifying gaps between organisational aspiration and patient experience.

Starting out as non-statutory bodies, PCNs have been slow to embrace patient representation. This is a significant missed opportunity, especially within the context of a drive to closer community integration. Representation in PCN decision-making forums could come from PPG members. Patient and provider representation including diverse VCS voices will strengthen PCNs, bringing a valuable array of views to decisions. Without these, PCNs, which have largely been led by primary care, will tend to revert to solving the problems of primary care rather than addressing the needs of their populations.

The next layer of patient involvement is the local Healthwatch, whose mission is to include the perspective of patients within decision-making, providing a reflective view of health services. As an independent statutory voice involved in discussions, the 'critical friend' role helps ensure patient voices are heard. This is also a frequent entry point for concerns raised about healthcare, providing an advocacy role on a system or individual level. Work on projects looking at patient experience of healthcare helps to focus attention on what is going well and what is not. Beyond this, health and wellbeing boards (HWBs) provide oversight of provision including social care and public health. HWBs are seen as partnership organisations rather than prime decision-makers, with a formal scrutiny role feeding back to providers.

There are many other groups who regularly interact with healthcare providers. The Care Quality Commission (CQC) and professional regulatory bodies provide oversight and regulation of healthcare systems and staff. Single-issue health charities often aim campaigns at GPs as well as funders, calling for more awareness and investment in specific parts of the healthcare system. Pharmaceutical representatives also target prescribers, knowing that money spent is more than repaid in prescriptions generated. Drug reps visiting physicians bring an almost double return on investment, while advertisements in medical journals which influence prescribing repay the cost five to one.[15] Private companies, always looking for ways to take on the more profitable parts of provision, vie for the attention of commissioners.

Health services have been slow to recognise the value of community resources. Avoiding signposting to community support may be due to lack of awareness, concern about boundaries or ceding organisational territory, but ends up professionalising care. Engaging relatives and volunteers to be directly involved in care improves the quality of care experienced, and grounds this as a function of community.

Volunteer involvement can add significant therapeutic value to a hospital stay. Helping with meals and drinks frees up nursing time and adds variety and companionship. Patients benefit from more intensive therapy than staff can provide, but simple chair-based exercises or games such as throwing and catching provide company, rebuild muscle and coordination, and are fun. Similarly, volunteers in clinics increase opportunities to socialise, improving the experience for attendees. Leg clubs provide companionship and a more social approach to people attending for dressing changes. Moving care closer to home, whether in peripheral clinics, community hospitals or outreach services, improves access to support and boosts local social capital.

Group consulting techniques reveal the expertise already within the community. Group-based consultations already work well for pain management and diabetes, but there are many other conditions that lend themselves to effective group-based support. Group consultations involve a clinician, a facilitator and a group of patients. Questions for the clinician are gathered in advance, and are discussed in front of the entire group. This increases the knowledge in the group, as many of the issues are common to attendees. Test results are shared, generating a strong motivation to improve results. Concerns about confidentiality are often unfounded, as patients are usually very happy to compare with others. Group models allow visiting specialists to offer longer consultations covering more detail while reaching more patients.

## Measuring the cost-effectiveness of care

Allocating care budgets means understanding where resources are most effectively invested. Spending should be based on best value, but this, of course, depends on what is meant by value. Commissioners need investment to generate savings somewhere else in the system, so an important part of the evidence base for interventions is the balance of cost to benefit. Calculating the cost of an input relative to the money saved by a better health outcome quantifies the cost-effectiveness of a health intervention.

Describing lives saved makes for an easy headline, but this metric is better defined as premature deaths prevented, as the bell still tolls for us all one day. Focusing on mortality distorts the picture somewhat, as this approach values a treatment that prevents a death but leaves someone fully dependent on care as equal to one that restored full health. Most people would not see this as of equal priority, so another metric was devised to account for this, the QALY (quality-adjusted life year). This attempts to value levels of dependency differently, in order to provide a measure by which success can be measured. QALYs are years in full health gained by an intervention, while DALYs (disability-adjusted life years) invert this to represent total years of life lost or lived with disability. Quantifying human life in this way carries insinuations, in particular a focus on function that implies that someone with disabilities has a lower value of life. Although the calculus of weighing remaining time against function is a decision patients may face, our perception of value changes as our circumstances do.

Using QALYs and DALYs as a metric helps to stratify provision of services towards those giving the most benefit for the funding available. The National Institute for Health and Care Excellence (NICE) threshold for funding is considered to be between £20,000 and £30,000 per QALY, though the presence of such a threshold is not confirmed by NICE. Decisions are more fluid, with refusal becoming more common towards the higher end of this threshold. The role of NICE is to judge the willingness of society to pay.[16]

As an example, one of the most cost-effective interventions available is help to stop smoking. The cost of nicotine replacement therapy per QALY gained by a smoker who successfully stops is under £2,000, a tenth of the NICE threshold, but cuts to local authority budgets have impacted on smoking cessation services, demonstrating how funding this through the most cash-strapped part of the system is a false economy. Meanwhile, some drugs are purchased at far higher cost relative to the benefit. The 2010 UK coalition government set up a £200 mn annual fund specifically for cancer drugs, which effectively increased the threshold to around £50,000 per QALY.[17] Spending higher amounts on particular diseases is inequitable, reinforces pharmacological approaches at the expense of other strategies, undermines the premise of NICE and reduces funding available for other conditions.

## Mental health services

The separation of services into physical and mental healthcare has continued the divide between mind and body into the way care is provided. Mental health services are arranged around tiers of treatment depending on acuity,

*Table 4.1* Tiered system of Mental Health services

| | |
|---|---|
| Tier 4 | Tertiary referral and inpatient units |
| Tier 3 | Specialist services such as CAMHS (Child and Adolescent Mental Health Service) and 'recovery' teams |
| Tier 2 | Targeted services such as primary mental health services, Youth Offending Teams and counselling (VCS or statutory, within or outside of education) |
| Tier 1 | Universal prevention by professionals such as GPs, health visitors, school nurses, teachers and social workers |
| Tier 0 | Not always included in models, but has been used to describe both self-help and user-led, peer-support models such as recovery colleges |

the degree of illness (Table 4.1). Services run in parallel to those for physical health, leaving gaps in provision for conditions which cross the divide. A patient with complex trauma, chronic pain and an eating disorder, for instance, may have three or more specialist teams involved, each treating only the part they consider their responsibility. Viewing a patient as a collection of tightly packaged diagnostic clusters ignores interactions between conditions, which unsurprisingly makes successful treatment much less likely.

Mental health services are usually run by different trusts from those running physical health services. This leads to huge boundary issues, causing problems as people fall through the gaps between overstretched services. Conditions where needs straddle traditional physical and mental provision of health require coordination rather than disjointed records, separate teams and services bristling with exclusion criteria.

Services can cause harm by intervening inappropriately for distress which can be better managed elsewhere. Medicalised solutions invite mutual dependency and disempower patients by assuming professional services are best placed to respond. Walls around teams force patients to climb over them to get help. Naming an urgent mental health response team a 'crisis team', for instance, invokes the idea of needing to be in crisis in order to access it. Professionals define access criteria to protect their capacity, but needing patients to be in crisis to offer help means interventions are always too late. This focus on reactive treatment has detracted from upstream work on prevention and wellbeing.

The recovery approach that prevails within mental health services defines expected outcomes for patients using tools such as the Recovery Star[18] to quantify aspects of living across ten outcomes measures. This approach neglects the effects of social determinants of health, locating problems within individuals rather than looking at how austerity and a decline in social capital have contributed to poor mental health. The activist collective Recovery in the Bin adapted the recovery star model to reflect the real precipitants of illness (Table 4.2).

*Table 4.2* Recovery and Unrecovery star measures[a,b]

| | |
|---|---|
| Recovery star | Managing mental health, physical health and self-care, living skills, social networks, work, relationships, addictive behaviour, responsibilities, identity and self-esteem, trust and hope |
| Unrecovery star | Poverty, loss of rights, unstable housing, sexism, transphobia and homophobia, discrimination, economic inequality, racism, trauma, loss of the welfare state |

Notes:
a MacKeith, Joy, Burns, Sara. *Mental Health Recovery Star*. Mental Health Providers Forum; 2009. https://www.centreformentalhealth.org.uk/sites/default/files/recovery_star_org_guide.pdf
b Recovery in the Bin. Unrecovery star. https://recoveryinthebin.org/

## Talking therapies

Psychological therapies within the NHS have predominantly been subsumed under the banner of Improving Access to Psychological Therapies (IAPT), a programme to make talking therapies more widely available. As the effectiveness of cognitive behavioural therapy (CBT) became clear, funding was diverted to expand provision, the intention being that the cost would be recouped from reductions in productivity losses and benefit claims.[19] An ambition for quantity means previous experience delivering psychological therapy is not necessary for new staff. The training of a psychological wellbeing practitioner (PWP) to deliver therapy according to the IAPT manual takes one day a week for a year, while working supervised.[20]

While CBT is undoubtedly effective for some, it does not suit all, and the reliance on one modality has left others harder to access. The specifications for delivery do not factor in the sharing of humanity that characterises effective therapeutic relationships. The style of group sessions tends to be didactic, and individual therapy was mostly by phone even before COVID-19 made this necessary. IAPT performance data suggests the program may not reach cost-effectiveness at £29,500 per QALY,[21] which is double the cost of adding antidepressants to usual care.[22]

IAPT services and many GPs use the PHQ-9 questionnaire to measure the severity of depressive symptoms. A focus on predominantly negative symptoms can be counter-productive in therapeutic consultations, ignoring strengths and medicalising distress into diagnoses of depression and anxiety. The widespread use of PHQ-9 and its counterpart for anxiety, the GAD-7, misses other narrative concerns which may be of far more significance to the patient, meaning that the score can misrepresent the experience of low mood symptoms.[23] Counting just those things that can be easily counted misses much relevant detail.

## Wider provision

Where and how could distress be better treated? Talking therapies and counselling are effective, but the capacity for one-to-one therapy is very limited.

Subsidiarity, acting at the lowest appropriate level, reduces the medicalisation of distress. Community development is both an up and a downstream intervention, providing resilience and addressing the consequences of trauma and marginalisation.

Other organisations providing alternatives to statutory services have an important role to play within mental health. Having access to alternative opinions helps to maintain choice and offer other views which may challenge medicalised concepts of health. The stigma of rejection and the possibility of different narratives around mental health mean that many people prefer to access support from VCS organisations, including peers who are 'experts in not being experts'.[24]

Peer support provides a way to democratise mental health, offering support by, rather than support for. This ranges from advocacy and mutual aid to peer-led support groups, which can be as effective as support from mental health professionals,[25] benefiting both patient and peer. Funding peer support reduces hospital readmissions,[26] paying for itself up to four times over.[27] Contributing lived experience, peer workers may be more effective than professionals in building self-esteem and engagement in the people they are working with.

Ensuring interventions address the determinants of health is the most effective way to improve outcomes. Five 'best buys' have been identified to improve mental health[28]:

- parenting skills supporting early years development
- lifelong learning, including health promotion in schools and ongoing education
- workplace interventions to improve working lives
- lifestyle and social changes
- community support and environment improvements

These all sit outside traditional healthcare provision, but are amenable to community-based interventions. Building social capital by connecting and nourishing what grows is a powerful generator of wellbeing and resilience against poor mental health. The human need for company, purpose and meaning is universal, and people lacking these are at greater risk of illness. Having someone to hear us and walk alongside us is hugely important for our health, but these roles are far better done outside of the healthcare system. Healthcare is good at identifying disease, but treating the underlying causes needs a community approach.

## Notes

Links and additional resources for this chapter can be found at www.communityhealth. uk/4-healthcare-structures

1  Marmot, Michael, Allen, Jessica, Goldblatt, Peter, et al. *Fair Society, Healthy Lives: The Marmot Review*. UCL; 2010. https://www.instituteofhealthequity.org/resources-reports/fair-society-healthy-lives-the-marmot-review

2 The public health budget (via local authorities) is £3.3 bn, hospitals cost £85 bn and GP practices, dentists and others £42 bn. Office for National Statistics. *Healthcare Expenditure, UK Health Accounts: 2019*. ONS; 2021. https://www.ons. gov.uk/peoplepopulationandcommunity/healthandsocialcare/healthcaresystem/ bulletins/ukhealthaccounts/2019

3 Coote, Anna, Penny, Joe. *The Wrong Medicine: A Review of the Impacts of NHS Reforms in England*. New Economics Foundation; 2014. https://neweconomics. org/2014/11/the-wrong-medicine/

4 Gray M, Airoldi M, Bevan G, McCulloch P. Deriving optimal value from each system. *J R Soc Med*. 2017;110(7):283–286. doi:10.1177/0141076817711090.

5 Jarman B, Gault S, Alves B, et al. Explaining differences in English hospital death rates using routinely collected data. *BMJ*. 1999;318(7197):1515–1520. doi:10.1136/ bmj.318.7197.1515.

6 Starfield, B, Shi, L, Macinko, J. Contribution of primary care to health systems and health. *Milbank Q*. 2005;83(3):457–502. doi:10.1111/j.1468-0009.2005.00409.

7 Dowrick C. Why do the O'Sheas consult so often? An exploration of complex family illness behaviour. *Soc Sci Med*. 1992;34(5):491–497. doi:10.1016/0277-9536(92)90204-4.

8 Regmi K, Mudyarabikwa O. A systematic review of the factors – barriers and enablers – affecting the implementation of clinical commissioning policy to reduce health inequalities in the National Health Service (NHS), UK. *Public Health*. 2020;186:271–282. doi:10.1016/j.puhe.2020.07.027.

9 Salway S, Mir G, Turner D, Ellison GTH, Carter L, Gerrish K. Obstacles to "race equality" in the English National Health Service: insights from the healthcare commissioning arena. *Soc Sci Med*. 2016;152:102–110. doi:10.1016/j.socscimed. 2016.01.031.

10 Smith R. Oh NHS, thou art sick. *BMJ*. 2002;324(7330):127–128. doi:10.1136/ bmj.324.7330.127.

11 See note 3.

12 Gerard K, Salisbury C, Street D, Pope C, Baxter H. Is fast access to general practice all that should matter? A discrete choice experiment of patients' preferences. *J Health Serv Res Policy*. 2008;13(suppl 2):3–10. doi:10.1258/jhsrp.2007.007087.

13 Russell, Cormac. We don't have a health problem, we have a village problem. In: *Community Medicine* Vol 1; 2020:1–12. https://www.nurturedevelopment.org/ wp-content/uploads/2018/09/we-dont-have-a-health-problem-we-have-a-village-problem8259.pdf

14 Oliver SR, Rees RW, Clarke-Jones L, et al. A multidimensional conceptual framework for analysing public involvement in health services research. *Health Expect*. 2008;11(1):72–84. doi:10.1111/j.1369-7625.2007.00476.x.

15 Gallan AS. Factors that influence physicians' prescribing of pharmaceuticals: a literature review. *J Pharm Mark Manage*. 2004;16(4):3–46. doi:10.3109/ J058v16n04_02.

16 Devlin N, Parkin D. Does NICE have a cost-effectiveness threshold and what other factors influence its decisions? A binary choice analysis. *Health Econ*. 2004;13(5):437–452. doi:10.1002/hec.864.

17 Chamberlain C, Collin SM, Stephens P, Donovan J, Bahl A, Hollingworth W. Does the cancer drugs fund lead to faster uptake of cost-effective drugs? A time-trend analysis comparing England and Wales. *Br J Cancer*. 2014;111(9):1693–1702. doi:10.1038/bjc.2014.86.

18 MacKeith, Joy, Burns, Sara. *Mental Health Recovery Star*. Mental Health Providers Forum; 2009. https://www.centreformentalhealth.org.uk/sites/default/ files/recovery_star_org_guide.pdf

19 Evans, Jules. A brief history of IAPT: the mass provision of CBT in the NHS. The History of Emotions Blog. Published May 30, 2013. https://emotionsblog. history.qmul.ac.uk/2013/05/a-brief-history-of-iapt-the-mass-provision-of-cbt-in-the-nhs/

20  National Collaborating Centre for Mental Health. The Improving Access to Psychological Therapies manual. Published online August 2021. https://www.england.nhs.uk/wp-content/uploads/2018/06/the-iapt-manual-v5.pdf

21  McCrone P. IAPT is probably not cost-effective. *Br J Psychiatry.* 2013;202(5): 383–383. doi:10.1192/bjp.202.5.383.

22  Kendrick T, Chatwin J, Dowrick C, et al. Randomised controlled trial to determine the clinical effectiveness and cost-effectiveness of selective serotonin reuptake inhibitors plus supportive care, versus supportive care alone, for mild to moderate depression with somatic symptoms in primary care: the THREAD (THREshold for AntiDepressant response) study. *Health Technol Assess.* 2009;13(22). doi:10.3310/hta13220.

23  Malpass A, Dowrick C, Gilbody S, et al. Usefulness of PHQ-9 in primary care to determine meaningful symptoms of low mood: a qualitative study. *Br J Gen Pract.* 2016;66(643):e78–e84. doi:10.3399/bjgp16X683473.

24  Repper J, Carter T. A review of the literature on peer support in mental health services. *J Ment Health.* 2011;20(4):392–411. doi:10.3109/09638237.2011.583947.

25  Mahlke CI, Krämer UM, Becker T, Bock T. Peer support in mental health services. *Curr Opin Psychiatry.* 2014;27(4):276–281. doi:10.1097/YCO. 0000000000000074.

26  See note 24.

27  Trachtenberg, Marija, Parsonage, Michael, Shepherd, Geoff, Boardman, Jed. *Peer Support in Mental Health Care: Is It Good Value for Money?* Centre for Mental Health; 2013. https://www.centreformentalhealth.org.uk/sites/default/files/2018-09/peer_support_value_for_money_2013.pdf

28  Friedli, Lynne, Parsonage, Michael. *Promoting Mental Health and Preventing Mental Illness: The Economic Case for Investment in Wales.* All Wales Mental Health Promotion Network; 2009.

# 5 Prescribing society

Presentations to healthcare cover the widest imaginable range of issues affecting the human condition, including distress and interpersonal issues. These manifest in many different forms, life events and circumstances always relevant. These 'social' problems are the main cause of attendance for around a fifth of GP appointments and contribute to many more.[1] These consultations about relationships, housing or employment cost around 5 per cent of the primary care budget.

Primary care has long been a convenient way for people to engage with statutory services. Family practitioners are trusted, familiar and accessible, and even when a problem is not primarily medical, the associated distress invokes the need for clinical review. This leaves clinicians managing everything from benefits advice to housing queries without the same skills or connections as teams set up to handle these. Signposting to the appropriate agencies still takes up an appointment. Healthcare is an expensive way to manage issues that can be better solved elsewhere. Lacking sufficient capacity to pick up this important but non-medical work, healthcare retreats into the familiarity of reactive medicine, treating the symptoms but missing the causes.

## Social prescribing

The recognition that many of the problems presenting to primary care are not medical in origin has led to the development of *social prescribing*, the use of non-medical sources of support. Innovative work, notably in Bromley-by-Bow,[2] pioneered social prescribers embedded into GP surgeries, supporting groups and demonstrating the benefits of reconnecting people with their community. This model has spread as the health improvement potential has become recognised. The real value of community health comes from creating and maintaining connections.

There is a need for help navigating systems, with welfare advice responsible for one in seven GP attendances.[3] Putting welfare advisors into surgeries reduces demand on healthcare.[4] The intricacies of referral pathways can render them impassable even for those used to working within the system. The sheer complexity of these structures generates complex responses (Conway's law). Someone who knows the way through the health and social care system

DOI: 10.4324/9781003391784-6

is a vital source of support. There may also be a need for advocacy, especially for those at the margins.

Another function is simply to be a witness to distress and life events. Many patients present without expectation that problems can be solved, but aware that sharing a problem makes it easier to bear. Standing alongside someone as their story plays is the privilege of health and care work, forging a deep knowledge of community. An ongoing relationship is the central component of care. People need to be heard, and anguish validated. Continuity, care and compassion should be at the heart of this.

## Social prescribers

A social prescriber is a non-clinical worker, usually based within a GP surgery, who spends time with patients exploring interventions outside of traditional healthcare. Variously known as social prescribers, community navigators, community connectors and link workers, these roles require a detailed knowledge of local community resources.[5] Social prescribing covers a wide spread of interventions, but the common factor is the non-clinical nature of encounters.

The most prevalent model still relies on gatekeeping by GPs, who identify social needs and either signpost directly or ask a social prescriber or link worker to get involved. Social prescribing is well received by patients, seen as less stigmatising than other interventions such as a counselling referral.[6] Discussion with social prescribers opens up options for non-clinical support, an alternative approach providing space for a different narrative to develop. Groups are often recommended, hosting activity which generates connections, peer support and improved sense of cohesion and meaning.

The idea of social prescribing is a laudable aim to reduce load on healthcare services by recognising when a problem could be dealt with more effectively elsewhere. Social prescribing opens up options to patient and practitioner, more time being especially useful when exploring other ways to manage distress.[7] Frequent attenders benefit from social prescribing approaches,[8] as isolation and health anxiety drive a significant proportion of attendances. Reductions in attendance for the most frequent users frees the most capacity; one fewer attendance each year for these patients would free up two days (1 per cent) of GP time.[9]

Social prescribing predominantly supports people in at-risk groups such as those with chronic illnesses or who are lonely or isolated, people with mental health problems and frequent attenders to primary care. People in marginalised groups in particular may find voluntary sector support more accessible than statutory services.[10]

Social prescribing can be a powerful way to address unmet needs on an individual basis. Much of that power comes from connections into multidisciplinary teams (MDT), with link workers part of a wellbeing team along with therapy, nursing and VCS. Social prescribers open the door to a wider range of health-creating interventions.

Social prescribing should not be a distraction from the loss of other assets, a new model of care to mask the loss of important community functions.[11] Public transport, for instance, is needed most by older residents, providing a social as well as transport function. Privatised bus routes that close for lack of profitability denude village and town alike. Diverting money into social prescribing while ignoring the basic social building blocks is a perverse outcome of different budget priorities. Social prescribing should not become a panacea to avoid addressing systemic problems.[12]

Organisations under tight financial restrictions have had little incentive to address issues on behalf of others. The ongoing internecine rift between health and social care has left large holes in society's safety net. The relentless reorganisation of the NHS has been to find ways to bypass these structural issues. Austerity budgets have led to the closure of much alternative provision, and cuts to preventative services have left problems more entrenched. Healthcare ends up catching those who have fallen through the holes, even when this is better done by others.

The complicated funding arrangements of care organisations have been the main hindrance to closer working at scale. The Better Care Fund (BCF) was introduced in 2013 as a way of diverting resources from health to social care, making projects addressing the joint overlap more feasible. Social care budgets had been cut drastically under the auspices of austerity, but the Cameron government had promised not to cut health expenditure, so the BCF became a way to divert funds towards other holes in the system, conveniently allowing money to be announced twice.[13] While the BCF has not been shown to provide value for money,[14] it has increased joint working to address some of the thorny problems lying in the gaps between organisations.

Currently a small social prescribing service is funded via primary care networks, but no money is allocated to supporting community interventions. The general principle within the NHS is that funding should follow the patient, though this stops abruptly at the edge of healthcare. Personal budgets are a potential route for funding to follow activity that sits outside traditional care provision. These offer a more flexible way to pay for alternative sources of care to improve outcomes that matter to patients. Assessments are based on self-chosen outcomes, and interventions paid for as part of an appropriate support plan agreed with the funding council. Most personal budget holders report improved self-esteem, dignity and sense of control.[15] However, personal budgets still rely on deficit-based assumptions and may reinforce consumerism within healthcare, opening up opportunities for privatisation.[16]

PCNs represent a new size of organisation, which better suits locality-based, cross-organisational care. This gives an opportunity for locally decided health priorities and outcomes that matter to the community. PCNs have a statutory duty to engage with health inequalities and better population health, and citizen input is a crucial part of this. Community representation counters the professionalisation of problems and the pull of serviceland.

Under the new PCN contract, social prescribing is now embedded within primary care, with a rapid rollout of link workers in GP surgeries.[17]

The advancement of social prescribing has somewhat preceded the evidence base, particularly regarding cost-effectiveness.[18] Despite this, social prescribing has multiplied, because the benefits are so apparent at individual level. How this translates into outcomes and value for money is less clear. The complexity of interactions and use of proxy outcome markers mean that estimates of cost-effectiveness vary widely, but social prescribing remains cheap in healthcare terms, especially for an important part of the interface at the edge of healthcare.

Social prescribing suits healthcare because it derives from the medical model; patients still expect and get a prescription, which opens up wider sources of support. Shifting interventions further upstream is good preventative medicine, but the process still medicalises the transaction. The model itself strongly reinforces the medical paradigm, whereby a second person asks a third to fix a problem with the first. Ensuring referrals go via GPs has appropriated community activity into healthcare, while defeating the purpose of reducing medical workload.

Many GPs feel unconfident in their information about sources of community support, and lack time to engage with social prescribing in already squeezed appointments.[19] Liability when signposting can still be a concern for clinicians, especially when going outside of statutory services. Recommendations, for example to get more exercise, do not carry liability, and some GPs prefer the use of the term 'referral' rather than 'prescription' for the same reason.[20] Regulatory advice is that doctors are not accountable for the actions and omissions of those to whom they have delegated care, although a decision to transfer care should be justifiable.[21]

There is no good reason why a probation worker, councillor or teacher should not have access to the same resources as the GP. Community assets being available to all saves diverting problems through healthcare. Opening access to social prescribing to other agencies demedicalises and lowers thresholds for accessing support. Multiple entry points equalise access to services.

Social prescribing works only if there is community activity to refer patients to, so needs to go hand-in-hand with community development, to ensure that communities themselves are able to be health-enabling. Fair access to funding for all providers would show that the VCS is not being used as a way to externalise costs. The current piecemeal VCS funding requires endless grant applications, usually from mutually supportive organisations competing for the same funding pot. Voluntary organisations have far better things to do than chase funding. A fair funding system that recognises the value in VCS provision would open up effective service provision.

A wide range of community resources available to social prescribing ensures diverse needs are met. A 'smörgåsbord' approach with a range of options to choose from seems to be the most effective strategy, as some activities will have particular resonance for some individuals. Most interventions are group-based, usually meeting regularly over a period of time. Groups may be based around a specific joint activity from which social aspects follow, or focus purely on bringing people together. Both approaches are valuable, the enhanced opportunity for socialisation being the common benefit.

*Table 5.1* Types of social prescribing[a]

| Signposting | Passing on information about sources of support |
| --- | --- |
| Light | Referrals for specific needs such as exercise or arts groups |
| Medium | A facilitator sees patients though referrals still based on specific needs |
| Holistic | Stronger links between practices and community groups addressing wider needs |

Note:
a Kimberlee R. What is social prescribing? *Adv Soc Sci Res J.* 2015;2(1). doi:10.14738/assrj.21.808.

Having a shared sense of purpose develops the sense of cohesion within a group, but the modality of a group matters less than the membership. From recovery colleges to Men's Sheds, the benefit of spending time with peers is unarguable. Groups offer opportunities for conversations that lead somewhere. Many of these connections are serendipitous, revealed while chatting, but the chance nature of these interactions seems to increase the quality of the relational changes they bring about.

Supporting group development lets statutory services encourage community development without prescribing the direction of travel. Providing regular training opportunities and a supportive infrastructure makes the setup and running of a group easier, so members can concentrate on the activities they enjoy. Much of the organisation needed is common to groups, and there is little point in each group writing their own safeguarding protocol, for instance, when these can be provided off the shelf for groups to adapt to their own needs. Back-office support lets groups focus on doing the things they do.

Just like individuals, organisations need resilience to adapt to changing situations. Groups are set up by enthusiasts, but energy can dissipate as time progresses and key members move away or health issues reduce attendance. Groups have a finite lifespan, but this transience should not be mourned, as ongoing needs will be picked up again. Where there is a gap to be filled, it may be a better use of resources to facilitate the startup of a new group than try to maintain one that is flagging. The strength of the VCS is in creativity and adaptability, evolving to meet changing needs. The bonds generated within groups survive as bridging ties that resurface elsewhere, bringing experience and new perspectives.

## Volunteering

Volunteering encompasses any helping activity without expectation of reward, whether formal (through organisations) or informal. Volunteers enjoy staying productive, taking an active role in society and the increased opportunity for interactions. Helping others is a strong motivation for volunteering, as well as gaining skills and work experience. Better social integration improves both the physical and mental health of volunteers.[22] Lower frailty and depression scores and better cognition, mental wellbeing and life satisfaction are all found in regular volunteers. Volunteers have lower mortality rates than non-volunteers, the effect becoming stronger with increased participation, although only for those taking part for altruistic (rather than personal) reasons.[23] Giving time lowers one's risk of mortality, but giving money does not, as this needs less commitment and generates no increase in social contact. Volunteering increases community resilience and connectedness.

Motivation, opportunity, time and other resources are necessary to get involved, but the actual trigger to start volunteering usually follows a particular event or catalyst.[24] Personal meaning in the proposed activity is important, but continued participation relies on the process being enjoyable and adequately resourced. If these factors are missing, stopping becomes more likely, although it is often a life event that brings a period of volunteering to an end.

Microvolunteering offers strictly time-limited ways to help, without any obligation for ongoing participation. This makes it easier for those with commitments such as employment or care responsibilities to take part. Microvolunteering is ideally suited to brief online activity, such as apps which allow sighted volunteers to help blind and visually impaired people via a live video call.[25] While virtual participation makes it feasible for those with mobility problems or living remotely to help, there is less interaction and sense of belonging with online volunteering. There is also a risk that 'slacktivism', online action supporting political or social causes, becomes a replacement for deeper engagement.[26]

Voluntary groups need organisers, who are typically volunteers themselves. Group organisers gain from being involved, but running groups often involves volunteers taking on multiple roles as others give them up. Getting pulled into extra roles creates role strain, which is a concern for some who would otherwise happily get involved. Processes lacking effectiveness and group dysfunction leading to cliques also put people off volunteering. Addressing these concerns and improving the quality of experience for participants keeps volunteers coming back.

Holding risk is a significant source of stress for volunteers. Working with people is always varied, and a significant disclosure or identification of a safeguarding concern is an ever-present possibility. People in voluntary roles may not feel confident about dealing with these issues, and the discomfort from feeling that one is holding excessive levels of risk threatens future participation. Practitioners are trained and supported to deal with this level of risk, but the same is often not true for volunteers. Support needs to be quickly accessible by prompt involvement of statutory services when needed.

A liaison role feeding back concerns to GPs helps providers to feel confident that risk is being managed. This role becomes the conduit between statutory and VCS services, sharing knowledge at patient, family and neighbourhood level. The wide overlap with safeguarding makes this an ideal role for a PCN safeguarding lead, who can attend multidisciplinary team and family network meetings. Providing this at PCN level makes the scale manageable, able to link people registered across different practices. Connections with the wider team mean concerns can quickly be raised with the appropriate professional. Teams who are often very quick to signpost patients to other organisations need to ensure they pick up referrals with the same alacrity. Why should signposting be one-way?

Healthcare under-recognises volunteers as a potential asset. The wider return from encouraging volunteers within the NHS recoups between three and ten times the investment.[27] Volunteer involvement can invoke concern about replacing paid staff, especially when taking on administrative roles, and should represent an addition to services, not a replacement. Volunteering is far less common with for-profit providers, which do not generate the same goodwill as public institutions. As market forces and competition become more pervasive within healthcare, loss of goodwill risks a loss of other assets.

## Directory of services

Every meeting discussing community resources reaches agreement that there is a real need for a better directory of local groups and assets. This usually follows on from the discovery of a new group or resource in conversation, and the recognition of how much activity there is to be aware of, even for those working within a community. It should be easy to know about the lunch clubs, yoga classes and all the other activities going on locally, but it is almost impossible for practitioners to keep track of all the various groups and activities that may be able to help the person in front of us. The networks that connect us are so complex and vast that we see only the threads that join to us, and even those who are most connected see only a fraction of what is going on locally. It is impossible to signpost without knowing the destination, so exploring assets within a community is important work.

Developing a map of assets shares knowledge and allows greater connectivity. Maintaining a comprehensive list is difficult, as questions immediately arise about entry criteria, aim, geography, sector, reach and audience. The relatively quick turnover of some groups together with short-term funding for pilot projects means that active review is needed to ensure details are up-to-date. Inadequate or wrong information quickly reduces engagement. When planning directories, there is a need to consider and decide on a number of issues to define reach and content:

- Who is this resource for? Is it just for professionals, and if so, why?
- Which activity should be included and which excluded? Is the scope for inclusion limited to statutory, VCS or private, and if so, why?
- How are these lists to be shared? If for wider use, what are the best mechanisms for ensuring access to those in need of the information?

A directory of community assets becomes a useful entry point for citizens to access services. Signposting on local authority websites tends to be the most reliable source of information. Clean navigation based around subject areas allows cross linking of services, to be accessible from different approaches.

The aim is to ensure people are able to access the right services initially. Duplication of assessment and effort is inefficient and expensive, so getting it right the first time is worthy of investment. Single point of access or 'no wrong door' type services provide a catchall for those who need help navigating the system. These should simplify access by collecting information for triage to the correct team.

## Referrals

Social prescribing interventions are seldom directly commissioned. In keeping with the reactive nature of healthcare, it is far more common for a group to approach health services with a view to partnership working. Budgets may require match funding from statutory organisations, meaning decision-makers need to recognise the value gained from interventions and be prepared to commit resources. This can be a source of strain, due to stretched budgets, unfamiliarity with VCS ways of working and the difficulty defining suitable outcome metrics on which to judge success. Demonstrating a causal improvement in outcomes is difficult, especially hard outcomes such as use of health care, morbidity and mortality. Concern that health spending may be perceived as being diverted to other activities is always present, as the case for interventions is not always well understood.

The referral process also needs consideration. Providing patients is the main function of health partners, who need to understand entry criteria. Referrers have a responsibility to ensure that onward referrals are appropriate and that suitable governance has been established. Some form of referral process is needed, gathering enough information for the receiving service to triage. This requires collecting contact details and understanding what input is needed. Referral data only need to be enough to decide on an initial pathway, without expecting others to do data collection on behalf of the receiving service. Direct access by self-referral empowers patients and ensures more accurate and person-centred information.

Groups tend to request similar information, including important medical issues, potential medication effects, safeguarding concerns and any other safety issues. A generic referral template is far preferable to services insisting on their own forms, which makes the process overly complicated for referrers. A detailed medical history is rarely necessary and indeed counterproductive when the aim is for non-medical support. The most useful question is to understand what the patient and referrer want to get from the referral.

Safety of participants needs to be considered, with emotional and psychological as well as physical risks addressed. Boundaries around sharing contact details and meeting up outside of groups should be considered, although participants will want autonomy to make these decisions for themselves. Routes for addressing issues and complaints should be clearly stated and safeguarding policies easily available, with named contacts for escalating concerns.

The common resource needs for groups are a space to meet in and a facilitator. Some activities such as singing or Tai Chi need very few external resources. Other activities such as pottery need access to expensive, specialist equipment, although commercial users might be happy to share. Meeting outdoors opens up suitable spaces that are free but dependent on the vagaries of weather. The COVID-19 pandemic has meant good ventilation is crucial, making the use of outdoor spaces safer for those at higher risk. A covered but well-ventilated outdoor space with access to toilets, transport links and somewhere to prepare drinks provides the widest utility.

## Assessing effectiveness

Understanding the effectiveness of an intervention depends on how effectiveness is judged. For health services, this may mean reduced demand, while patient-oriented metrics will focus on a far wider range of outcomes that matter to individuals. Wellbeing scores are commonly used to show improvements. Patient Reported Outcome Measures (PROMs) are more directly health-oriented tools, which help to measure interventions but may miss individual priorities. Breaking outcomes into discrete targets loses the holistic aspect that people find valuable, the uniqueness and complexity of each individual narrative lost when forced into boxes for the purposes of measurement.

What is notable throughout the literature around social prescribing interventions is the lack of good quality evidence proving the benefits. There is weak evidence that social prescribing reduces demand on healthcare services. One review found emergency department attendances and demand for GP services were reduced by a quarter in those referred to social prescribing.[28] Improvements in loneliness, isolation and better mental and physical health have also been shown.[29] There are gains in self-esteem and wellbeing for patients, but GP workload is not reduced.[30] The qualitative benefits of the experience are clear to attendees, but far less often has this been translated into robust arguments that these interventions are worthwhile in healthcare terms. Short follow-up periods, missing control groups, varied outcome measures and the use of proxy markers all make it harder to show benefit.

The ordinary magic of writing groups or parkrun may become tarnished when seen as a prescription rather than something enjoyable to do for its own sake. Quantifying the benefits helps to allocate resources appropriately. A linear relationship between interventions and outcomes should not be assumed,[31] as the interactions between these dynamic factors may not show a direct causal relationship. Interpretation of outcomes needs to consider the complexity of such systems.

While research is often considered a specialist skill, assessing the benefit of an intervention is feasible without specialist knowledge. The priority is to collect appropriate data at the time. Providing a control group is the best way to assess the difference an intervention makes, by randomly allocating people to an intervention or alternative, typically 'usual care'. Local ethics committees and universities are good sources of advice on study design.

*Table 5.2* Common Outcomes Framework for social prescribing[a]

| | |
|---|---|
| Individual | ONS4 wellbeing score |
| | Patient Activation Measure |
| Community | Referrals received |
| | Coping with demand |
| | Potential capacity |
| | Volunteer numbers |
| | Gaps in provision |
| | Development needs |
| Health and social care system | GP appointments |
| | ED attendances |
| | Inpatient bed days |
| | Prescriptions |
| | Staff morale |

Note:
a NHS England. *Social Prescribing and Community-Based Support: Summary Guide*; 2020. https://www.england.nhs.uk/publication/social-prescribing-and-community-based-support-summary-guide/

Quality of life questionnaires such as EQ-5D[32] and the positively worded WEMWBS [33] are accessible, validated and well recognised within the literature. Wider data on health care use are helpful for commissioners, who are under pressure to reduce healthcare spending and need to show value. Collecting information such as GP appointment usage or NHS number is more complex, but allows more accurate measuring of healthcare use.

A Common Outcomes Framework has been developed in an attempt to standardise assessment.[34] This covers the impacts of social prescribing on the person, on community groups and on the health and social care system. Suggested goals for individuals are around being more connected, more physically active, coping better and feeling in control. Community groups are asked about demand, capacity, gaps and development needs.[35] The system impacts that can be most easily quantified look at healthcare use across primary and secondary care. Consistent coding within GP records counts referrals, although this again reinforces the route of going via GPs, risking recording capacity rather than demand.

Individual wellbeing and patient activation measures (PAM) are suggested for social prescribers to use for each new referral.[36] The ONS4[37] asks people to score four factors out of ten: how happy they feel, how anxious, how satisfied with life and whether the things they do are worthwhile. The PAM tool records people's confidence to manage their health and wellbeing themselves. These measures do not cover outcomes such as connections, physical activity or sense of community, for which data are not routinely captured at individual level.

## Social return on investment

Assessing the cost effectiveness of models that have impacts across a system should reflect the wider benefits, including the social value gained. Social return on investment (SROI) measurement attempts to capture the costs and benefits of an intervention across multiple sectors.[38] Financial value is attributed to inputs and outputs, with some assumptions necessary, for instance valuing volunteer time at national minimum wage, or putting a value on environmental impact. When the improved social value of community-based approaches is taken into account, using SROI helps to level the playing field between extractive and co-operative funding bids.

The SROI process identifies stakeholders and builds an impact map detailing resources and outcomes. Outcomes need to have a value attributed, including 'deadweight' activity that would have happened anyway as a result of other factors. This helps to adjust for the lack of an appropriate control group, which is often impractical given the unique and complex nature of the systems being assessed. Value displaced from elsewhere should be included, as well as future impact, reduced demand on services and the potential drop-off in activity seen in many projects over time. SROI is a proxy financial value, without the robustness to provide meaningful comparison with other SROIs.

Return on investment is the ratio of net value created to value of investment:

$$ROI = \frac{gain - cost}{cost}$$

A ratio of zero is cost neutral, meaning that gains are the same as the cost, while a ratio of one means that an extra pound is saved for every pound spent. Employing a community development worker gives an SROI of 2.16, meaning extra social value of just over twice the investment is created within the community group. Including the extra value brought by participating volunteers brings a return of almost six to one. However, most of the value gained is outside of the project, with the wider local community gaining fifteen times the value of the original investment. A third of this extra value created comes from improved supportive relationships, and over a quarter from increased trust and sense of belonging.[39]

Corporate social responsibility includes social and environmental factors when making decisions. The Public Services (Social Value) Act 2012 requires all public sector procurement decisions to consider these aspects. Counting the social, environmental and economic value is also known as *triple bottom line* accounting, which counts not just the financial aspects but assesses the impact on people, planet and prosperity. This helps to integrate provision of services within a framework that values the effects on local communities.[40]

Making links across communities improves health within those communities. There is a need for asset maps and connectors. Groups and volunteering are both health-enabling, and those benefits can be realised by developing community and connections. Exploring the different modalities groups are based on shows how these benefits manifest. Connecting, staying active, noticing, learning, and giving are all health-enabling.

## Notes

Links and additional resources for this chapter can be found at www.communityhealth.uk/5-prescribing-society

1 Caper, Kathleen, Plunkett, James. *A Very General Practice: How Much Time Do GPs Spend on Issues Other Than Health?* Citizens Advice Bureaux; 2015. https://www.citizensadvice.org.uk/Global/CitizensAdvice/Public%20services%20publications/CitizensAdvice_AVeryGeneralPractice_May2015.pdf
2 Bromley by Bow Centre. https://www.bbbc.org.uk/
3 Social Prescribing Network. *Report of the Annual Social Prescribing Network Conference.* University of Westminster; 2016. https://www.artshealthresources.org.uk/wp-content/uploads/2017/01/2016-Social-Prescribing-Network-First-Conference-Report.pdf
4 Krska J, Palmer S, Dalzell-Brown A, Nicholl P. Evaluation of welfare advice in primary care: effect on practice workload and prescribing for mental health. *Prim Health Care Res Dev.* 2013;14(03):307–314. doi:10.1017/S1463423612000461.
5 Drinkwater C, Wildman J, Moffatt S. Social prescribing. *BMJ.* Published online 2018:l1285. doi:10.1136/bmj.l1285.
6 Bertotti M, Frostick C, Hutt P, Sohanpal R, Carnes D. A realist evaluation of social prescribing: an exploration into the context and mechanisms underpinning a pathway linking primary care with the voluntary sector. *Prim Health Care Res Dev.* 2017;19(03):232–245. doi:10.1017/s1463423617000706.
7 Friedli, Lynne, Vincent, Ashley, Woodhouse, Amy. *Developing Social Prescribing and Community Referrals for Mental Health in Scotland.* Scottish Development Centre for Mental Health; 2007. https://www.artshealthresources.org.uk/docs/developing-social-prescribing-and-community-referrals-for-mental-health-in-scotland/
8 Friedli, Lynne, Jackson, Catherine, Abernethy, Hilary, Stansfield, Jude. *Social Prescribing for Mental Health - a Guide to Commissioning and Delivery.* CSIP North West Social Prescribing Development Project; 2008. https://citizen-network.org/library/social-prescribing-for-mental-health.html
9 Heywood P. An assessment of the attributes of frequent attenders to general practice. *Fam Pract.* 1998;15(3):198–204. doi:10.1093/fampra/15.3.198.
10 See note 8.
11 Salisbury H. Social prescribing and the No 17 bus. *BMJ.* 2019;364. doi:10.1136/bmj.l271.
12 See note 5.
13 Williams, David. The better care fund will soon be redundant. *Health Serv J.* Published online October 2, 2015. https://www.hsj.co.uk/the-bedpan/the-better-care-fund-will-soon-be-redundant/5090830.article
14 National Audit Office. *Health and Social Care Integration.* Department of Health, Department for Communities and Local Government and NHS England; 2017. https://www.nao.org.uk/wp-content/uploads/2017/02/Health-and-social-care-integration.pdf
15 Hatton, Chris. *Personal Health Budget Holders and Family Carers: The POET Surveys 2015.* Think Local Act Personal; 2015. https://www.thinklocalactpersonal.org.uk/_assets/Resources/SDS/POETPHB2015FINAL.pdf
16 Ferguson I. Increasing user choice or privatizing risk? The antinomies of personalization. *Br J Soc Work.* 2007;37(3):387–403. doi:10.1093/bjsw/bcm016.
17 Baird, Becky, Lamming, Laura, Bhatt, Ree'Thee, Beech, Jake, Dale, Veronica. *Integrating Additional Roles into Primary Care Networks.* The King's Fund; 2022. https://www.kingsfund.org.uk/sites/default/files/2022-02/Integrating%20additional%20roles%20in%20general%20practice%20report%28web%29.pdf
18 Buck, David, Ewbank, Leo. *What Is Social Prescribing?* The King's Fund; 2020. https://www.kingsfund.org.uk/publications/social-prescribing

19 See note 6.
20 Kimberlee, Richard. *Developing a Social Prescribing Approach for Bristol.* University of the West of England; 2013. https://uwe-repository.worktribe.com/output/927254
21 General Medical Council. Delegation and referral. https://www.gmc-uk.org/ethical-guidance/ethical-guidance-for-doctors/delegation-and-referral
22 Mundle C, Naylor C, Buck D. *Volunteering in Health and Care in England: A Summary of Key Literature.* The King's Fund; 2012. https://www.kingsfund.org.uk/sites/default/files/field/field_related_document/volunteering-in-health-literature-review-kingsfund-mar13.pdf
23 Konrath S, Fuhrel-Forbis A, Lou A, Brown S. Motives for volunteering are associated with mortality risk in older adults. *Health Psychol.* 2012;31(1):87–96. doi:10.1037/a0025226.
24 Brodie Ellen, Hughes Tim, Jochum V, Miller S, Ockenden N, Warburton D. *Pathways through Participation: What Creates and Sustains Active Citizenship?* Pathways through participation; 2011. https://involve.org.uk/sites/default/files/uploads/Pathways-Through-Participation-final-report_Final_20110913.pdf
25 Be My Eyes. See the world together. https://www.bemyeyes.com/
26 Heley J, Yarker S, Jones L. Volunteering in the bath? The rise of microvolunteering and implications for policy. *Policy Stud.* 2022;43(1):76–89. doi:10.1080/01442872.2019.1645324.
27 Teasdale S. *In Good Health: Assessing the Impact of Volunteering in the NHS.* Institute for Volunteering Research; 2008. https://www.bl.uk/collection-items/in-good-health-assessing-the-impact-of-volunteering-in-the-nhs
28 A 28 per cent reduction in demand for GP services, 24 per cent reduction in emergency department attendances. Polley M, Bertotti M, Kimberlee R, Pilkington K, Refsum C. *A Review of the Evidence Assessing Impact of Social Prescribing on Healthcare Demand and Cost Implications.* University of Westminster; 2017. https://www.researchgate.net/publication/318826738_A_review_of_the_evidence_assessing_impact_of_social_prescribing_on_healthcare_demand_and_cost_implications
29 Bickerdike L, Booth A, Wilson PM, Farley K, Wright K. Social prescribing: less rhetoric and more reality. A systematic review of the evidence. *BMJ Open.* 2017;7(4):e013384. doi:10.1136/bmjopen-2016-013384.
30 Loftus AM, McCauley F, McCarron MO. Impact of social prescribing on general practice workload and polypharmacy. *Public Health.* 2017;148:96–101. doi:10.1016/j.puhe.2017.03.010.
31 Daly, Sorcha, Allen, Jessica. *Voluntary Sector Action on the Social Determinants of Health.* Institute of Health Equity; 2017. https://www.instituteofhealthequity.org/resources-reports/voluntary-sector-action-on-the-social-determinants-of-health
32 EQ-5D. https://euroqol.org/
33 Tennant R, Hiller L, Fishwick R, et al. The Warwick-Edinburgh Mental Well-being Scale (WEMWBS): development and UK validation. *Health Qual Life Outcomes.* 2007;5(1):63. doi:10.1186/1477-7525-5-63.
34 NHS England. *Social Prescribing and Community-Based Support: Summary Guide*; 2020. https://www.england.nhs.uk/publication/social-prescribing-and-community-based-support-summary-guide/
35 NHS England. *Social Prescribing Link Workers: Reference Guide for Primary Care Networks – Technical Annex*; 2020. https://www.england.nhs.uk/publication/social-prescribing-link-workers-reference-guide-for-primary-care-networks-technical-annex/
36 See note 35.
37 Office for National Statistics. Personal well-being user guidance. Published online September 26, 2018. https://www.ons.gov.uk/peoplepopulationandcommunity/wellbeing/methodologies/personalwellbeingsurveyuserguide

38  Nicholls, Jeremy, Lawlor, Eilis, Neitzert, Eva, Goodspeed, Tim. *A Guide to Social Return on Investment*. Cabinet Office: Office of the Third Sector; 2009. https://neweconomics.org/2009/05/guide-social-return-investment/

39  NEF Consulting. *Catalysts for Community Action and Investment: A Social Return on Investment Analysis of Community Development Work Based on a Common Outcomes Framework*. Community Development Foundation; 2010:58. https://socialvalueuk.org/report/catalysts-for-community-action-and-investment-sroi/

40  Jones, Naomi, Yeo, Alice. *Community Business and the Social Value Act*. Power to Change; 2017. https://www.powertochange.org.uk/wp-content/uploads/2017/08/Report-8-Community-Business-Social-Value-Act.pdf

# 6 Social prescriptions

Many people feel disconnected from others around them. The health impacts of disconnection are profound, affecting quality of life and leading to illness and premature mortality. Communities create health by increasing opportunities to connect. Building social connections provides individual and community resilience through bridging links, skills acquisition and time spent with others. Community assets are a rich source of health-enabling activity, ranging from creating spaces and opportunities to more multifaceted interventions.

There is such breadth and diversity of community activity that no single overview of how the strands interweave could be possible or meaningful. We connect to others in myriad ways. These connections are most powerful when the things we enjoy interact with social capital, activity and nature.

## Faith groups

For much of our history, religious worship has been the main reason for coming together regularly, and faith groups remain a substantial part of associational life for many people. In more oppressive societies, places of worship have often been relatively spared from prohibitions on gatherings, especially where political power is allied with a particular religious group. A steady shift towards a more secular society has seen church attendances in the UK more than halved since 1980.[1] Sport and entertainment events attract far larger congregations now.

Having a religious belief is associated with better self-reported health.[2] Volunteers actively engaged in public religious practices describe better physical and mental health.[3] This applies less to those with belief who do not attend, who miss out on the effects on social cohesion and the reinforcement of shared norms and values within the group. Faith groups remain a vital part of community activity, with strong ethoses and links. Service to others is fundamental within most faiths, though how this manifests varies.

There is sometimes caution within healthcare about signposting to faith organisations, in part due to concerns about the professional overlap with religion. Regulator guidance about spirituality states that care should not be offered to further a particular political or religious view, and makes clear that

DOI: 10.4324/9781003391784-7

a practitioner's belief should not cause distress to others, but otherwise says nothing about services provided by faith groups. The outward manifestation of actions is what people experience, not the beliefs behind them.

Collaboration between local faith groups recognises that combining resources benefits all. Mutual respect between faiths makes shared working more feasible, though projects are more typically run by one group rather than several. A degree of competition between groups can be stimulating, motivated by seeing the work of others. Collaboration is to be welcomed, but when given a challenge, having a defined project bonds groups. Projects should represent shared community values and actively seek engagement from across a community.

## Exercise and activity

Inactivity and obesity are, along with smoking, responsible for the largest burden of lives lost prematurely. Inactivity leads to one in six deaths in the UK, costing the NHS £1 bn annually.[4] Increasing activity is the most effective way to improve our health, with even small increases in activity bringing significant reductions in risk of death and disease. Promoting activity is hugely cost-effective medicine.

Extolling the therapeutic and preventative value of activity has a long history, going back to Hippocrates (460–370 BCE) and Galen (129–216 CE), who both prescribed exercise.[5] This has long represented a safer alternative to more interventional medical treatment. Over time, the role of advocating physical education slowly shifted from medicine to schools and sports coaching, developing a focus on competition, which left the less athletic behind.

Originally known as medical gymnastics, physiotherapy began as a profession in 1894. The need for rehabilitation of wounded soldiers and patients with polio developed the medical use of massage and exercises to develop strength and coordination. Bed rest is harmful for most conditions, and early mobilisation is crucial to prevent deconditioning. Specialist rehabilitation skills extend to group-based work for conditions such as falls and Parkinson's disease.

Many of us spend much of our lives in very similar positions, which lets stabilising muscles weaken and joints lose their full range of movement. Stretching improves suppleness, while building core stability, the supportive muscle tone which protects our joints, can help to prevent musculoskeletal problems. Yoga and Pilates are accessible ways to improve tone and stability. Strengthening exercises are as important as aerobic ones to maintain health or rehabilitate following illness. An hour a week of muscle strengthening exercise reduces mortality by up to 20 per cent.[6]

Approximately 4 million people fall each year in the UK, one in three of those aged sixty-five and over, and one in two of those aged eighty and above. As well as the mortality and fracture risk from falls, confidence is dramatically affected, leading to more limited activity and horizons, a poorer quality of life, and an increased risk of social isolation. Tai Chi, a Chinese martial art for mind and body, reduces the risk of falls by up to a third, comparing well with other exercise.[7] This is ideally suited to group work, as happens in China, where many people practise together in public parks. Tai Chi can be adapted to be a seated activity, accessible to people with dementia and cognitive impairment.

Our increasingly sedentary lifestyles have made it only too clear how important aerobic activity is for our health. Inactivity causes more than 35,000 deaths annually in the UK.[8] Half an hour of moderate activity five times a week reduces mortality by a fifth.[9] Increasing activity beyond this reduces mortality further, but the most benefit comes from gentle increases from sedentary levels of activity.

Activity is also important for our mental health. Exercise is as effective as psychotherapy and medication for depression,[10] at lower cost and without the same side effects. This is partly physiological, but exercise also improves self-esteem and opportunities for socialisation.

The words *exercise* and *activity* carry different connotations. The term *activity* is more encompassing, including many actions that increase heart rate but may not be considered as exercise. Exercise can imply a formal element, which can be off-putting for some, while sport similarly can bring unwelcome associations with competition. The value and health benefit is across all forms of activity.

UK guidance for adults is to aim for two and a half hours a week of moderate activity, or an hour a day for children and young people.[11] Activity such as cycling or brisk walking is considered of moderate intensity. Vigorous activity such as running brings the same benefits in half the time, or even shorter spells of very vigorous activity, such as sprinting or climbing stairs.

*Table 6.1* Activity

| | |
|---|---|
| Activity | 30 minutes of moderate activity five times a week reduces mortality from all causes by 19 per cent. Increasing this to an hour of moderate activity daily reduces mortality by a further 5 per cent.[a] |
| Walking | Walking improves fitness and cardiovascular parameters such as blood pressure, cholesterol and body mass, reducing risk of coronary heart disease by 6 per cent and stroke by 15 per cent.[b] Walking for Health programs costs £3,775 per QALY, with a return on investment of 3.36.[c] |
| Falls | Falls cost the NHS more than £2.3 bn annually.[d] |

Notes:
a Woodcock J, Franco OH, Orsini N, Roberts I. Non-vigorous physical activity and all-cause mortality: systematic review and meta-analysis of cohort studies. *Int J Epidemiol.* 2011;40(1):121–138. doi:10.1093/ije/dyq104.
b Hanson S, Jones A. Is there evidence that walking groups have health benefits? A systematic review and meta-analysis. *Br J Sports Med.* 2015;49(11):710–715. doi:10.1136/bjsports-2014-094157.
c France, Jonathan, Sennett, James, Jones, Andy, et al. *Evaluation of Walking for Health: Final Report to Macmillan and the Ramblers.* University of East Anglia, Ecorys; 2016:191.
d National Institute for Health and Care Excellence. *Falls in Older People: Assessing Risk and Prevention.* NICE; 2013. https://www.nice.org.uk/Guidance/CG161

Physical activity includes housework, active travel and recreation as well as exercise. Breathing rates need to increase, even if only slightly, to get benefit. Around two-thirds of UK adults achieve this level of activity, but a quarter of adults manage less than half an hour of activity in a week.[12] Women are less likely to be active than men, and activity also reduces with increasing age, disability or unemployment.

The phrase 'exercise on prescription' describes clinical recommendations ranging from suggestions in passing to increase activity to making exercise referrals. Health professionals who are themselves more physically active tend to refer more into exercise on prescription schemes, personal experience making their advice more credible. Asking about activity encourages uptake. The General Practice Physical Activity Questionnaire (GPPAQ)[13] is a validated and quick metric stratifying people into four levels of activity: inactive, moderately inactive, moderately active and active. Brief advice is effective enough that offering it wherever possible is worthwhile. Known as Making Every Contact Count (MECC), even thirty seconds of advice and opportunistic signposting helps to open up new avenues of support without nagging.

Barriers to engagement include the perception of a need for specialist clothing, which puts participation out of reach for some financially. A supportive environment for exercise and schemes to encourage beginners increases participation. Running has one of the lowest entry requirements of any activity, needing only a suitable pair of shoes and a supportive bra for women, which reduces discomfort and may improve performance. The Couch to 5K app is an accessible way to start running, consisting of a nine-week program of audio recordings narrating thirty minute walks. Running is gently introduced for increasing lengths of time to build up stamina and fitness until participants are able to run for the duration. Couch to 5K groups are mutually supportive and often linked to existing running clubs.

parkrun (always spelt as one word, lowercase) is the most widely known form of group exercise. parkrun is a weekly, free, timed five-kilometre run or walk, starting at 9 a.m. local time on Saturday. Beginning in 2004 as a time trial in a park with a few friends, parkrun is now worldwide. There have been 40 million finishes across nearly eight hundred parkruns in the UK. Junior parkrun is a shorter two-kilometre run for four- to fourteen-year-olds and their families on a Sunday morning. Normalising exercise for children encourages their families to become more active as well.

All parkruns are volunteer led, with a national organisation handling governance and the infrastructure connecting times to runners. The timed aspect is an important part of the experience, and provides useful feedback on performance. Walkers are most welcome to parkwalk, and need not be put off by the word 'run' in the title. One of the volunteer roles is to be 'tailwalker', following at the end to ensure that no participant comes last. The only thing needed to join a parkrun is a free, downloadable barcode. A briefing before the start establishes a sense of shared purpose. Visitors are welcomed, and milestones are celebrated. The chance to stay on for a drink and a chat

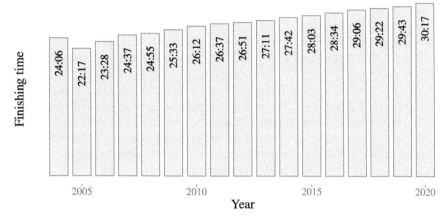

*Figure 6.1* Average finish times at parkrun, UK.

afterwards opens up the opportunity for interactions. These abundant brief contacts make parkrun 'community adhesive'.[14]

Pleasingly, average parkrun finish times have steadily increased (Figure 6.1), showing how parkrun has been taken up by less-fit individuals. An increase in average times at the local parkrun would be a good aspiration for PCNs aiming to increase activity in their populations.

There are also economic benefits to local hospitality and leisure as 'tourists' enjoy visiting other parkruns, often planning trips with a parkrun attendance in mind. The various parkrun clubs celebrate achievements such as volunteering or completing a particular number of runs. These reinforce the feeling of investment and sense of identification, which keeps people coming back.

---

**Box 6.1   Ross-on-Wye parkrun**

Ross-on-Wye parkrun started in 2019, sparked by a question on the town message board. The local running group provided the expertise with support from the two local GP surgeries. Planning meetings were held at one surgery in the evenings. There was a wide knowledge of local assets among the group, with connections into businesses, council and health. Ross was the first parkrun to have GP practice involvement from the start, and the hundredth parkrun to be part of the Royal College of General Practitioners (RCGP) parkrun practice initiative.

From the first meeting to launch took around nine months. Finding the funding was the main factor slowing progress. A mix of personal donations and sponsorship from local businesses reached the target to buy the equipment. Half the cost was match-funded from parkrun UK.

As the health benefits of the extra exercise would have been recouped within the first fortnight,[15] funding should have been more forthcoming. PCNs are now better placed to be supporting local health-enabling activity.

The planning needed included permissions and risk assessments. A takeover of a neighbouring parkrun helped build confidence before the launch date in August 2019. Inaugural parkruns can attract large crowds, so promotion was kept local to keep numbers manageable for a new team. Local GP practices signpost patients looking to get more active towards parkrun, and parkwalkers are strongly encouraged.

The course encircles playing fields in a lovely setting next to the river, with the sports centre café open afterwards for coffee, cake and a catch-up. parkrun has been a huge success, with good local engagement and a group of regular volunteers, but not without missing some weeks. The problem with a riverside course is the river, the course taking weeks to settle after floods. Celebrating the heritage of the region, an alternative course takes in nearby orchards, courtesy of a local cider maker. parkrun generates a steady stream of 'tourists' who travel to attend different events, contributing to the local economy.

Another accessible way to exercise in company is to join a walking group, offering activity combined with conversation across a wide range of fitness levels. Providing good infrastructure increases participation. Maintaining plentiful and accessible routes leading to greenspace is an investment in our health. The Walking for Health partnership with GP practices supports patient groups to exercise. Some groups such as Mental Health Mates focus on mental health and peer support.[16] Beat the Street is a challenge which gamifies walking to school,[17] awarding points for exploring the local area, which can motivate at individual, group and school level.

The health and social capital shared exercise generates is impressive, but many other sports also offer camaraderie, teamwork and purposeful physical activity. From rowing and rugby to dominos and darts, having a shared focus is enough to gain the benefits of group cohesion. Spending time with trusted adults outside of immediate family or caregivers provides important role models for young people. Exposure to the protective behaviour of trusted adults is particularly crucial for those without stable home environments. Regular sports participation in childhood increases resilience, and the benefit of participating in sports clubs or community groups persists into adulthood, halving rates of mental illness in participants with four or more adverse childhood experiences.[18]

The intensity of activity is quantified as MET (metabolic equivalent of task), which equates to one calorie per kilogram of bodyweight per hour. Moderate activity such as leisurely cycling has an estimated MET rate of

*Table 6.2* QALY gains from activity[a,b]

| Activity | METs | Minutes | Example activity | Annual QALYs gain when done weekly | Years to gain one QALY |
|---|---|---|---|---|---|
| Walking | 3.5 | 60 | Walking for an hour | 0.0187 | 53.5 |
| Cycling (leisurely) | 4 | 150 | Cycling 15 mins to work and back, five days a week | 0.0534 | 18.7 |
| Cycling (vigorous) | 10 | 45 | 45-minute bike ride | 0.0400 | 25.0 |
| Gardening | 3.8 | 180 | An afternoon gardening | 0.0609 | 16.4 |
| Swimming | 10.3 | 40 | Swimming 50 laps | 0.0367 | 27.3 |
| Rowing | 5.8 | 60 | An hour rowing | 0.0310 | 32.3 |
| Sailing | 3.3 | 180 | Three hours sailing | 0.0528 | 18.9 |
| Running | 9.8 | 30 | Weekly parkrun | 0.0262 | 38.2 |

Notes:
a Ainsworth, BE, Haskell, WL, Herrmann, SD, et al. *The Compendium of Physical Activities Tracking Guide*. Healthy Lifestyles Research Center, College of Nursing & Health Innovation; 2022. https://sites.google.com/site/compendiumofphysicalactivities/
b Papathanasopoulou E, White MP, Hattam C, Lannin A, Harvey A, Spencer A. Valuing the health benefits of physical activities in the marine environment and their importance for marine spatial planning. *Mar Policy*. 2016;63:144–152. doi:10.1016/j.marpol.2015.10.009.

around 4,[19] so an hour of cycling adds up to four MET hours (Table 6.2). Each MET hour of activity increases lifespan by nearly an hour (54 minutes, 0.00010265 of a year),[20] making each MET hour worth around £2 at the NICE threshold for cost per QALY.

These numbers imply a level of precision that is rather more than the rough estimate they are, but they still give an idea of the magnitude of the effect. Running for half an hour at a MET of 9.8 works out at 4.9 MET hours. At 54 minutes gained per MET hour, this adds 264 minutes to life, adding up to an extra year of life after doing a weekly parkrun for 38 years. The effect is not linear, as the benefits of exercise are most for the least active and tail off with further increases in activity, but quantifying activity in this way shows how the time and intensity of exercise contribute to health.

The actual activity prescribed often matters far less than the excuse it provides to be in a restoring environment. There is strong evidence that being outdoors brings health benefits, and environments rich in nature seem to have independent health-promoting properties. Sunshine on our skin helps our immune system and protects against osteoporosis. Productive gardening such as allotmenting keeps people active and produces seasonal, locally grown, cheap food of high nutritional value. 'Green exercise' combines ecological benefits and an opportunity for shared outdoor exercise. Whether litter picking or tree planting, the direct environmental benefit also rewards volunteers, while making use of energy that would otherwise be turning a treadmill. As with other social prescriptions, it is important to acknowledge the risk of commodifying nature when 'prescribing' it as something to be consumed, rather than it being an innate part of our lives.

## Nature

Those who work with groups will recognise that connections are more easily made when outdoors. Any formality felt sitting in halls and meeting rooms disappears when people get together outside. Anyone who has sat around a campfire will be familiar with how the setting changes the nature of the conversation. There is something about a closer interaction with nature that acts as a great leveller, allowing more authentic conversations and more potent connections. Individuals who are more connected to nature show better functioning, improved wellbeing and personal growth.[21] Increased connectedness improves stress responses, with improvements in sleep quality and duration after spending time in greenspace.[22]

Exposure to greenspace has been shown to have wide-ranging health benefits including reduced mortality.[23] People with access to greenspace are more likely to be physically active, improving health and saving healthcare costs. Perceived health is better in those with greener environments near to their homes,[24] especially for young and elderly people and those in lower socioeconomic groups. Children spending time in nature at an early age avoid 'nature-deficit disorder'[25] and are far more likely to enjoy nature as adults.[26] People who move to a greener area have improved mental health,[27] better quality greenspace improving health more.[28] The association between greenspace access and health is less pronounced in higher-income areas, where private gardens are a substitute. The inequality in mortality ascribed to income deprivation is lowest in the greenest areas, suggesting a protective effect of greenspace, which seems to modulate the effects of inequality in the same way that social cohesion does.

Including nature in clinical environments is beneficial; surgical patients with a view of trees have shorter hospital stays and need less pain control than those whose windows look out onto a brick wall.[29] Stress recovery theory (Roger Ulrich)[30] explains how exposure to nature reduces physiological changes and markers of stress. There is a strong evolutionary component, with humans primed to respond positively to natural environments that are favourable to survival, even though our needs are now met in very different ways. An innate need to consider potential for food, water and survival still seems to make some environments resonate for us. Across different cultures there is a strong preference for trees and landscapes that resemble those of the African savanna,[31] even for people with no prior knowledge of these. Biophilia is part of our evolutionary heritage, an innate affiliation humans have for other life forms,[32] which subverts our attempts at independence from the natural world.

Being in natural environments is refreshing because it changes our attention. Directed attention requires continued focus on a task and is fatiguing, leading to distractions and inefficient performance. Being in nature, watching wildlife or listening to music inspires effortless indirect attention known as fascination. 'Hard' fascination, such as watching sport or playing computer games, does not allow the space for reflection that the 'soft' fascination of nature provides. The theory of attention restoration (Stephen Kaplan)[33] suggests that it is the very complexity of natural vistas that allows our minds to refocus and restore. Complex patterns in nature are too detailed for us to be able to process, and this overloading of our processing abilities seems to refresh our focus. There are parallels with the use of stimulants to treat ADHD, and indeed children with ADHD show improved attention after spending time in natural environments.[34] To be effective, environments need to be different to the spaces we normally inhabit, and have enough 'extent' to suggest another possible world, rich and diverse.

## Blue prescribing

Views of water provide constantly changing patterns, which seem to be particularly effective in restoring attention, the characteristic soundscape of water also contributing to the experience. Being on or in the water connects us with the elements, engendering respect for nature while giving a different perspective looking back to shore. Two-thirds of adults say that being near water improves their mental health.[35]

Blue prescribing refers to activities around water. There are historical medical associations with bathing in water, which has been prescribed since the eighteenth century, spa and seaside towns thriving as visitors came to 'take the waters'. Cold water swimming lowers blood pressure, reduces stress hormones and improves immune function and mood.[36] Immersing the face in cold water stimulates a 'diving response' which improves cerebral blood flow. Swimming in these conditions carries risks from cold water shock, hypothermia and afterdrop, a further loss of central heat after swimming due to rapid rewarming, so needs acclimatisation and care. Water can reduce the impact of disability, for example hydrotherapy or diving, though it also brings extra considerations for safety of participants.

Aquatic activities in the UK such as sailing, angling and canoeing are popular forms of exercise. Water also brings more diverse exposure to nature, watching wildlife being a favourite pastime. Interacting with wildlife when participating in wetland nature-based interventions leads to clinically significant improvements in wellbeing and anxiety scores.[37]

*Table 6.3* Health benefits of being outdoors

| | |
|---|---|
| Greenspace | Access to greenspace increases physical activity by 24 per cent, which would save the NHS £2.1 bn annually if everyone in England had similar access.[a] |
| | Access to greenspace reduces mortality, improves cholesterol and reduces the incidence of type 2 diabetes.[b] |
| | There are 1.2 billion visits annually to natural environments in England annually, gaining 110,000 QALYs with a value of £2.2 bn.[c] |
| Wildlife | Volunteering with wildlife programmes has an SROI of up to 8.50.[d] |
| Blue prescribing | Activity in aquatic environments saves 24,853 QALYs annually, worth £176 mn.[e] |

Notes

a Stone, Dave. *An Estimate of the Economic and Health Value and Cost Effectiveness of the Expanded WHI Scheme 2009*. Natural England; 2013. doi.org/10.13140/RG.2.1.4190.4720.

b Twohig-Bennett C, Jones A. The health benefits of the great outdoors: a systematic review and meta-analysis of greenspace exposure and health outcomes. *Environ Res.* 2018;166:628–637. doi:10.1016/j.envres.2018.06.030.

c White MP, Elliott LR, Taylor T, et al. Recreational physical activity in natural environments and implications for health: a population based cross-sectional study in England. *Prev Med.* 2016;91:383–388. doi:10.1016/j.ypmed.2016.08.023.

d Bagnall, Anne-Marie, Freeman, Charlotte, Southby, Kris, Brymer, Eric. *Social Return on Investment Analysis of the Health and Wellbeing Impacts of Wildlife Trust Programmes.* The Wildlife Trusts; 2019. https://www.wildlifetrusts.org/sites/default/files/2019-09/SROI%20 Report%20FINAL%20-%20DIGITAL.pdf

e Papathanasopoulou E, White MP, Hattam C, Lannin A, Harvey A, Spencer A. Valuing the health benefits of physical activities in the marine environment and their importance for marine spatial planning. *Mar Policy*. 2016;63:144–152. doi:10.1016/j.marpol.2015.10.009.

## Green therapies

Mindfulness and talking therapies work well in natural environments. The woodland setting for forest bathing, Shinrin Yoku, enables CBT to treat depression more effectively.[38] There are similarities with eye movement desensitisation and reprocessing therapy (EMDR), which is used to treat the effects of trauma. Both work by encouraging reflection in a controlled environment.

Bringing nature into care environments helps, with indoor plants and natural sounds improving the wellbeing of staff and patients. Playing birdsong and showing natural images reduces agitation during personal care in care home residents with advanced dementia.[39] Behavioural interventions incorporating nature can reduce the use of pharmacological treatments, saving £70 mn and improving outcomes.[40]

People with dementia show increased wellbeing after spending time outdoors, especially in natural environments. Wander gardens in residential settings improve mood and quality of life and reduce agitation and medication use among people with dementia.[41] Carer concern can be an issue; four-fifths of carers believe dementia impairs the ability to be outdoors, whereas only one-fifth of people with dementia agree.[42] Gardening groups increase wellbeing scores in people with early-onset dementia, with better sense of belonging, time orientation and more talking points in conversation.[43]

Mixing nature and therapy is not new. Modern medicines developed from herbal cures grown in physic gardens and hedgerows. Sanatoria offered a countryside cure for people with tuberculosis. Gardens are reflective spaces which encourage mindful awareness. The hospice movement is closely associated with gardens, which provide space for the inevitable reflection on mortality that end-of-life care invokes.[44] Gardening is an accessible and therapeutic way to be closer to nature and spend time outside, increasing physical activity and wellbeing and reducing stress hormones.[45] Window boxes and indoor plants bring the benefits of horticulture into homes without gardens.

**Food and nutrition**

Community gardening offers growing space to those without access to a garden, providing company, habitat for wildlife and fresh seasonal local food. Sense of belonging is strengthened by undertaking tasks together. Community gardening brings the most wellbeing benefit to people in individualistic societies, who have less of a culture of shared community working.[46] This 'agresistance' rejects the corporatisation of food production in favour of environmental justice.[47] Gardening spaces reduce inequality by including people with cognitive impairment and physical disabilities. Working with the earth reframes the marginalised as 'active, expert, capable and productive community workers / members'.[48]

---

**Box 6.2  Ross community garden**

Ross community garden was established in 2013 with funding from a local soft fruit company. Growing areas are available to people without access to land, supported by a horticulturalist and other volunteers. A plot of land central to the town is both a haven for nature and a relaxed and friendly place to spend time. Schools and other groups use the facilities, which include polytunnels providing ventilated shelter from the elements. A Zero Waste stall reduces food waste by making available excess produce from supermarkets and distribution chains. Nutritious food is available to all for free, donations accepted from those able to pay. Framing this as an initiative to reduce food waste reduces the stigma of needing help.

---

Poor nutrition costs the NHS an estimated £6 bn annually, mainly due to higher levels of cardiovascular disease and cancer.[49] Fruit and vegetables are very good for us, each extra portion reducing the chance of coronary heart disease by 4 per cent.[50] Cheap food is of poor quality, meaning that diet is an important factor driving health outcomes worsened by inequality.

*Table 6.4* Food and nutrition

| | |
|---|---|
| Poor nutrition | £6 bn annual NHS cost, 10 per cent of DALYs lost.[a] |
| Food banks | UK food distributions have increased by 60 times since 2009. 2.5 million emergency food parcels were given out in 2020–21.[b] |
| Food waste | 9.5 million tonnes of food were wasted in the UK in 2018, 69 kg per person.[c] |
| | UK food waste generates 25 million tonnes of greenhouse gases.[c] |

Notes:
a Rayner M. The burden of food related ill health in the UK. *J Epidemiol Community Health.* 2005;59(12):1054–1057. doi:10.1136/jech.2005.036491.
b Tyler, Gloria. *Food Banks in the UK.* House of Commons Library; 2021:31. https://researchbriefings.files.parliament.uk/documents/CBP-8585/CBP-8585.pdf
c WRAP. *Food Surplus and Waste in the UK – Key Facts.* Waste and Resources Action Programme; 2020:16. https://wrap.org.uk/sites/default/files/2020-11/Food-surplus-and-waste-in-the-UK-key-facts-Jan-2020.pdf

Teaching of nutrition in schools remains undervalued, and many young people leave home lacking cooking skills. Teaching people to cook is an effective way to improve nutrition. Many people would benefit from the opportunity to learn to cook, to be able to access affordable and nutritious food. Lower-income diabetic patients living in 'food deserts' in the US who were taught how to cook showed improved blood pressure and cholesterol.[51] The experience of people who have done it before is a powerful community asset.

Health problems from poor quality food are now exacerbated by hunger, illustrated starkly by the rise of food banks over the last decade, now numbering well over two thousand in the UK. People seek help due to poverty and adverse life experiences, having exhausted support from others. While the generosity of communities keeps food banks open, much food is still wasted. Zero-waste food stalls provide an outlet for unsold food that would otherwise be tipped. Community fridges are a convenient way to share or swap excess produce. Supermarket demands for high cosmetic standards leave some of each harvest perfectly usable but unsellable through usual distribution chains. Known as 'gleaning', produce in fields that would otherwise be wasted can be rescued by volunteers who are allowed to pick anything suitable left after the main crop has been harvested. Gleaning provides good sources of local, seasonal nutrition for food banks and local distribution.

## Learning

Ongoing learning helps stimulate and preserve cognitive function. Engaging with adult learning increases civic participation and exposes learners to a wider range of people, improving diversity of relationships.[52] Healthy behaviours such as exercise increase in adult learners, along with the likelihood of stopping smoking. Schools and colleges have accessible spaces which are ideally suited to group work and are often available outside normal working hours.

---

**Box 6.3    Cervical cancer educational project**

Involving educational organisations in health promotion projects is an effective way of spreading messages, giving students gain real world experience, building skills and connections. Working with Healthwatch, the local sixth-form college designed a cervical cancer awareness campaign. Delivery of the message was more effective having been designed by students of similar age to those the campaign was aiming to reach. The project generated discussion and knowledge about recognising signs of the disease, forming a community asset of health information disseminated to family members and friends.

---

Ongoing learning throughout our lives is very good for our wellbeing. Much of our social identity and sense of meaning is bound up in our work roles, meaning that retirement can be a source of loss, opportunities for interactions drastically reduced as bonding ties turn to bridges. While much thought goes into financial planning for retirement, the social aspects of leaving the workplace are usually neglected. Retirees have much to give, and communities benefit from the time and skills available. Retired people also gain from the opportunity and stimulation of teaching and disseminating the vast knowledge acquired from a lifetime of work. Clubs such as the University of the Third Age (u3a)[53] provide opportunities to share interests and generate discussion for a positive later life.

Older men are particularly at risk from isolation after retirement. Men have a life expectancy three years less than women[54] and are less likely to seek help with health issues. Isolation and loneliness are significant risk factors for suicide, rates being three times higher for men than women,[55] so creating opportunities for socialisation that address the specific needs of older men is even more important.

Men's Sheds provide a place for older men to connect, create and chat. There are around six hundred Sheds in the UK, offering a combined work and social space, sharing a workshop and company. Most 'Shedders' are retired, and have found attending a Shed rekindles a sense of community and of purpose previously fulfilled through the workplace. Repairing or working on a variety of projects, Sheds can help with maintenance of community assets. The lack of hierarchy is an important factor, with members' experience valued equally. The informality and lack of a boss is appreciated by attendees, who have no need of pressure to hit targets, enjoying instead a workplace in which a chat over coffee is just as important as working.

One important decision for Sheds concerns inclusion of those with cognitive problems. Power tools present a safety risk, which inevitably generates worries about insurance and liability. Some Sheds admit women, but there are also Women's Sheds fulfilling a similar function. The gendered nature of the interventions may be an important component to the benefits, related to

differences in the way people of the same gender interact; men may communicate better 'shoulder-to-shoulder' than face-to-face.[56]

Attending Sheds increases activity, benefitting mental health and wellbeing, mainly via social inclusion, which reduces isolation.[57] Dissemination of
skills and a heightened sense of purpose increase feelings of self-worth.[58]
Although good for health, encouraging attendance at Men's Sheds for the
health benefit may be counterproductive, and a 'health-by-stealth' approach
is more likely to be effective.[59]

Repair cafés, originating in the Netherlands, have a related function.
People bring broken things to pop-up cafés for volunteers to help fix, the
person bringing the object actively involved in repairing it. This feeds a circular economy, reducing waste and emissions, a visible example of sustainable
practice with wider impacts. Each product repaired saves up to 24 kilograms
of greenhouse gases,[60] making a significant difference across the two thousand repair cafés worldwide. Volunteers' experience is supported by a database of repair techniques, though a legal right to repair would help most to
counter the extractive and wasteful nature of built-in obsolescence.

## Mentoring

Not everyone leaves school with the skills to manage in a workplace.
Opportunities for further development are sparse for the one in ten young
people not in education, employment or training, some of whom have had
significant exposure to adverse experiences. Access to benefits is vulnerable
for school leavers who disengage. Mentoring can be an important intervention, particularly for those at risk of overlap with the criminal justice system. Apprenticeships provide adult role models and the dissemination of
skills. Young people gain great benefit from a stable role model outside of
the family, especially where this is lacking in the household. Demonstrating
ways of being as an adult, in particular promoting positive examples of mas-
culinity, is helpful for younger men. It takes a whole village to raise a resilient child.

Intergenerational mixing is a powerful way of improving cultural cohesion
and diversity. Mentoring is one way to provide this, along with shared intergenerational housing and other projects mixing younger and older people.
Spending time with adults outside of the family helps children become familiar with a wider range of people, and also benefits the adults. People with
dementia are able to help preschool age children with activities, showing
increased positive behaviours when children are present.[61]

## Arts and creativity

Creative endeavours help us to explore wider questions about our place in
the world. The arts consist of 'everything you don't have to do',[62] which are

often the things that give our lives meaning. The health potential of arts can come both from appreciating and creating art. The power of art to move us is well recognised; people can be overwhelmed by an artwork (Stendhal syndrome).[63]

Arts embedded within health settings usually sit within one of these roles.[64]

- art and design within the healthcare built environment
- visual and other art forms to improve the environment for patients, visitors and staff
- medical humanities for teaching communication skills to clinicians
- psychotherapy using art
- community groups using art for wellbeing

Medical humanities enhance communication skills using art and literature to rehumanise medicine by considering what really matters. By focusing on the words that patients use as well as the medical problems they represent, clinicians can explore a wider narrative than the narrow seam of symptoms that medical training concentrates on.

The media we consume influence our health beliefs. The narratives we use to understand and talk about illness come predominantly from media portrayals. Drama, films, books, music and opera teach about the basic human condition, reflecting and reinforcing cultural and linguistic norms. Versions of the same stories have been told in thousands of consulting rooms to generations of doctors.

The creative use of art within health is already established in the work of art therapists. Usually found within mental health teams, art therapy uses art as a medium for psychotherapy, drawing out emotional issues with visual imagery. The creative process has far wider benefits than this, and makes an excellent core activity for a group, stimulating the flow of conversation during a session. There is a powerful sense of achievement from making something, and combining this with socialisation is an effective mix. Crafts express joy in the creation of things we need. Decoration and artistic expression add to our cultural heritage, helping to create a shared social identity.

Arts-for-health projects need a protected space for making new things, which encourages participation and creativity, playfulness and improvisation.[65] Play is an important part of learning, giving permission to experiment and get things wrong. Equal status between facilitator and participants breaks down hierarchies.

Arts on Prescription (also known as Arts on Referral) brings wellbeing benefits to participants, especially for women, older people and those from lower socioeconomic groups.[66] Those participating show a heightened sense of empowerment, as well as benefits to mental health and social inclusion.[67] Participating in art projects reduces healthcare use and costs.[68] The sharing of experiences is what underlies the wellbeing improvements.[69]

---

**Box 6.4   Poetry group**

Ledbury Poetry Festival funded a surgery creative writing group, open to all patients and facilitated by a poet. The group met fortnightly in a room at the GP surgery, writing poetry on themes chosen by the members. Strong bonds were formed, participants socialising and supporting each other. They enjoyed trips to literature festivals, published anthologies of their work and continued to meet for years after the project officially ended.

---

**Bibliotherapy**

Bibliotherapy refers to the therapeutic use of literature for health. This takes different forms, from self-help books to creative writing groups. Books on Prescription schemes aim to make psychological interventions much more widely available.[70] Books focused on health problems are made available through public libraries, sometimes 'prescribed' by a clinician. These books can be used as an adjunct to therapy or as a standalone resource. Books on Prescription provide accessible, trusted information and convenient access to CBT approaches.

Novels give insight into the human condition. Stories bring perspective and open up new possibilities. Librarians and booksellers are good sources of recommendations, as are lists of suitable novels as literary remedies.[71] Discussion at book groups establishes and evolves social norms. For young people, books can provide words and opportunities to be able to express feelings. The Junior Books on Prescription list[72] gives a way for children and their caregivers to explore subjects for which words can be hard to find, helping to 'give sorrow words'.[73] Discussing how the protagonist in a story coped can be a helpful and less threatening way to address issues vicariously.

The Human Library[74] offers people instead of books. People with expertise in the effects of marginalisation offer their time for discussion of topics in a safe space, challenging views and stereotypes and reducing stigma.

Our Books on Prescription service was set up in 2012 in collaboration with the county library service. This provided copies of self-help books across county libraries, mostly based on CBT principles. A separate shelf near the entrance promotes the books to those browsing. Books were chosen from a wide range of self-help books to be accessible and reliable sources of advice. A one-page document with a brief description of each book is available for GPs and other referrers to give to patients.

Writing even briefly about salient personal experiences improves physical and mental health and reduces doctor visits.[75] Writing about imaginary trauma gives a similar level of benefit, but not for people with PTSD or those who start with a story that is already formed. Constructing stories helps the writer to consider the external perspectives of potential readers. This involves arranging the narrative into a coherent order, which adds structure and meaning, helping to reach resolution. Working through explanations for events makes them easier to deal with.

## Music

Choirs and musical ensembles form a pure expression of communal creativity, producing something far more than the sum of its parts. As with nature, pleasure in experiencing music seems to be innate to humans. Participating in music also has wellbeing benefits. Older adults randomised to join a choir had fewer doctor appointments, fewer falls, less loneliness and better morale compared with a control group.[76] Medication use was less for the choral group, whose participation in activities increased, remaining so one year later.

The wide range of muscular activity involved in singing is likely to be particularly beneficial for some conditions. The abnormal stride cadence of Parkinson's disease improves after singing songs with strong rhythmic content. The parts of the brain stimulated by music are relatively spared in dementia, allowing music to be enjoyed regardless of levels of cognitive function. Participating in music stimulates memory and bonding and reduces behavioural and psychological symptoms of dementia.[77]

Learning and practising techniques for diaphragmatic breathing helps to maintain lung function in people with chronic respiratory disease. Patients with lung disease who join a singing group have fewer symptoms[78] and better respiratory function,[79] though the main benefit comes through group membership. Participants report positive feelings of joy, self-belief and structure in life from attending regularly, as well as the achievement from building up to a performance.[80]

## Prescribing social capital

There is a far wider social capital that all these interventions bring. Connections continue outside of groups, bringing together participants who would otherwise be at risk of isolation. The actual focus of the group is what leads people to join, but the social benefits happen irrespective of the group modality. Finding the right level of challenge in an activity that has personal salience increases enjoyment, which leads to ongoing participation.

Social prescribing interventions provide a degree of challenge in an environment shared with others. Resilience comes through broadened social networks and improved skills and confidence, with far-reaching social capital gains. Connections to others add meaning and importance, reducing self-destructive impulses and providing a buffer against adverse events. Sense of coherence (Aaron Antonovsky) [81] comes from the confidence that internal and external environments are predictable, that resources to deal with challenges are available, and that engagement is worthwhile. Our sense of coherence is shaped by consistency, having a voice in decisions, and an appropriate level of challenge.

A person's ability to cope with stress comes from events having meaning, comprehensibility and manageability. Agreeing with others about meaning leads to cognitive consonance, a congruent view of the world as 'making sense'. In the salutogenic model, this in turn facilitates coping strategies, known as *generalised resistance resources*. Comprehensibility describes how understandable internal and external stimuli are perceived to be. Manageability reflects the availability of resources. Combining these creates our sense of coherence. These factors have influence at collective as well as individual level, meaning that sense of coherence can be a feature of organisations as well as people.

Self-efficacy, belief in one's ability to perform a task, is enhanced not just by performing and practising, but through watching others.[82] This modelling encourages belief in individual capabilities and allows the development of new behaviour patterns. Exposure to challenges desensitises arousal and relaxes physiological states. The confidence that arises from an achievement is transferable to other skills and situations. This stands in contrast to learned helplessness, where the perception of lack of control induces passivity, particularly in those whose loci of control are more external.[83]

## Flow

As well as the social benefits of participation, there is a strong individual component. Learning something new pushes ourselves, expanding repertoires within our self-identity. Competitive traits become subsumed in a challenge to become better versions of ourselves. Change starts to happen when we push at the edge of our identities. Just as antidepressants work by shifting to an alternative viewpoint, stretching our self-identity enables reflection. The roots of the word 'ecstasy', *ex - stasis*, refer to standing outside of one's self. Providing this additional perspective is a crucial part of any therapeutic intervention.

Manual, creative work allows time for this. There are times within these endeavours where one's sense of self gets lost, caught up within the moment. Known as *flow* (Mihaly Csikszentmihalyi),[84] the feeling of complete absorption in an activity is transcendent. Doing an activity for the sake of it and enjoying the challenge lets us live within the moment. People report an altered sense of time during flow, the linear time of *chronos* giving way to *kairos*, time experienced as moments rather than minutes. Focused dissociation leads to a loss of self-consciousness as the separation between task and performer fades, relieving anxiety.

Flow is most likely when the level of challenge is equal to the level of skill, which is the optimal state for learning. High skill and low challenge leads to boredom, while the opposite increases anxiety. The motivation to master a skill is an important evolutionary strategy. The rewards foster a drive to replicate the experience, developing skills further. Pushing ourselves to learn new skills seems to be innate, but we need opportunities to allow this expression, to find our own flow.

## Notes

Links and additional resources for this chapter can be found at www.communityhealth. uk/6-social-prescriptions

1 British Religion in Numbers. Church attendance in Britain, 1980–2015. http:// www.brin.ac.uk/figures/church-attendance-in-britain-1980-2015
2 Office for National Statistics. *Religion and Health in England and Wales: February 2020. Analysis of a Range of Health Outcomes of People of Different Religious Identities in England and Wales.* ONS; 2020. https://www.ons.gov.uk/people populationandcommunity/culturalidentity/religion/articles/religionandhealth inenglandandwales/february2020/pdf
3 McDougle L, Handy F, Konrath S, Walk M. Health outcomes and volunteering: the moderating role of religiosity. *Soc Indic Res.* 2014;117(2):337–351. doi:10.1007/ s11205-013-0336-5.
4 Office for Health Improvement and Disparities. Physical activity: applying All Our Health. Published online March 10, 2022. https://www.gov.uk/government/ publications/physical-activity-applying-all-our-health
5 Berryman JW. Exercise is medicine: a historical perspective. *Curr Sports Med Rep.* 2010;9(4). https://journals.lww.com/acsm-csmr/Fulltext/2010/07000/Exercise_is_ Medicine__A_Historical_Perspective.7.aspx
6 Momma H, Kawakami R, Honda T, Sawada SS. Muscle-strengthening activities are associated with lower risk and mortality in major non-communicable diseases: a systematic review and meta-analysis of cohort studies. *Br J Sports Med.* Published online February 28, 2022:bjsports-2021–105061. doi:10.1136/bjsports-2021-105061.
7 Nyman SR. Tai Chi for the prevention of falls among older adults: a critical analysis of the evidence. *J Aging Phys Act.* 2021;29(2):343–352. doi:10.1123/ japa.2020-0155.
8 Allender S, Foster C, Scarborough P, Rayner M. The burden of physical activity-related ill health in the UK. *J Epidemiol Community Health.* 2007;61(4):344–348. doi:10.1136/jech.2006.050807.
9 Woodcock J, Franco OH, Orsini N, Roberts I. Non-vigorous physical activity and all-cause mortality: systematic review and meta-analysis of cohort studies. *Int J Epidemiol.* 2011;40(1):121–138. doi:10.1093/ije/dyq104.
10 Cooney GM, Dwan K, Greig CA, et al. Exercise for depression. Cochrane Common Mental Disorders Group, ed. *Cochrane Database Syst Rev.* Published online September 12, 2013. doi:10.1002/14651858.CD004366.pub6.
11 See note 4.
12 Sport England. *Active Lives Adult Survey*; 2020. https://bit.ly/CCH6_activeLives
13 Department of Health and Social Care. General practice physical activity questionnaire (GPPAQ). https://www.gov.uk/government/publications/general-practice-physical-activity-questionnaire-gppaq
14 Tobin, Simon. parkrun is community adhesive. parkrun UK Blog. Published May 23, 2022. https://blog.parkrun.com/uk/2022/05/23/parkrun-is-community-adhesive/
15 Assuming a MET of 4, $\times$ 100 people $\times$ 2 weeks $\times$ 0.00010265 = 0.082 QALYS which is thirty days. At the lower threshold of NICE willingness to pay, this is worth £40,000. One hundred people starting running or walking a parkrun weekly gains two years of life annually.
16 Mental Health Mates. Peer support & community. Walking & talking for your mental health. https://www.mentalhealthmates.co.uk/

17  Public Health England. Beat the Street: getting communities moving. https://www.gov.uk/government/case-studies/beat-the-street-getting-communities-moving

18  Hughes K, Ford K, Davies AR, Homolova Lucia, Bellis MA. *Sources of Resilience and Their Moderating Relationships with Harms from Adverse Childhood Experiences. Report 1: Mental Illness.* Public Health Wales NHS Trust; 2018. https://core.ac.uk/download/pdf/186465916.pdf

19  Ainsworth, BE, Haskell, WL, Herrmann, SD, et al. *The Compendium of Physical Activities Tracking Guide.* Healthy Lifestyles Research Center, College of Nursing & Health Innovation; 2022. https://sites.google.com/site/compendiumofphysical activities/

20  Papathanasopoulou E, White MP, Hattam C, Lannin A, Harvey A, Spencer A. Valuing the health benefits of physical activities in the marine environment and their importance for marine spatial planning. *Mar Policy.* 2016;63:144–152. doi:10.1016/j.marpol.2015.10.009.

21  Pritchard A, Richardson M, Sheffield D, McEwan K. The relationship between nature connectedness and eudaimonic well-being: a meta-analysis. *J Happiness Stud.* 2020;21(3):1145–1167. doi:10.1007/s10902-019-00118-6.

22  Shin JC, Parab KV, An R, Grigsby-Toussaint DS. Greenspace exposure and sleep: a systematic review. *Environ Res.* 2020;182:109081. doi:10.1016/j.envres. 2019.109081.

23  Twohig-Bennett C, Jones A. The health benefits of the great outdoors: A systematic review and meta-analysis of greenspace exposure and health outcomes. *Environ Res.* 2018;166:628–637. doi:10.1016/j.envres.2018.06.030.

24  Maas J, Verheij RA, Groenewegen PP, de Vries S, Spreeuwenberg P. Green space, urbanity, and health: how strong is the relation? *J Epidemiol Community Health.* 2006;60(7):587–592. doi:10.1136/jech.2005.043125.

25  Louv R. *Last Child in the Woods: Saving Our Children from Nature-Deficit Disorder.* Algonquin Books of Chapel Hill; 2008.

26  Wood CJ, Smyth N. The health impact of nature exposure and green exercise across the life course: a pilot study. *Int J Environ Health Res.* 2020;30(2):226–235. doi:10.1080/09603123.2019.1593327.

27  Alcock I, White MP, Wheeler BW, Fleming LE, Depledge MH. Longitudinal effects on mental health of moving to greener and less green urban areas. *Environ Sci Technol.* 2014;48(2):1247–1255. doi:10.1021/es403688w.

28  Mitchell R, Popham F. Effect of exposure to natural environment on health inequalities: an observational population study. *The Lancet.* 2008;372(9650): 1655–1660. doi:10.1016/S0140-6736(08)61689-X.

29  Ulrich RS. View through a window may influence recovery from surgery. *Science.* 1984;224(4647):420–421. doi:10.1126/science.6143402.

30  Ulrich RS, Simons RF, Losito BD, Fiorito E, Miles MA, Zelson M. Stress recovery during exposure to natural and urban environments. *J Environ Psychol.* 1991;11(3):201–230. doi:10.1016/S0272-4944(05)80184-7.

31  Bird, William. *Natural Thinking: Investigating the Links between the Natural Environment, Biodiversity and Mental Health.* RSPB; 2007. https://www.ltl.org.uk/wp-content/uploads/2019/02/natural-thinking.pdf

32  Wilson EO. *Biophilia: The Human Bond with Other Species.* Harvard Univ. Press; 1994.

33  Kaplan S. The restorative benefits of nature: toward an integrative framework. *J Environ Psychol.* 1995;15(3):169–182. doi:10.1016/0272-4944(95)90001-2.

34  Taylor AF, Kuo FE, Sullivan WC. Coping with ADD: the surprising connection to green play settings. *Environ Behav.* 2001;33(1):54–77. doi:10.1177/00139160121972864.

35  Mental Health Foundation. *Nature. How Connecting with Nature Benefits Our Mental Health.* Mental Health Awareness Week 2021. https://www.mentalhealth.org.uk/sites/default/files/2022-06/MHAW21-Nature-research-report.pdf

36 Knechtle B, Waśkiewicz Z, Sousa CV, Hill L, Nikolaidis PT. Cold water swimming—benefits and risks: a narrative review. *Int J Environ Res Public Health.* 2020;17(23):8984. doi:10.3390/ijerph17238984.

37 Maund, Irvine, Reeves, et al. Wetlands for wellbeing: piloting a nature-based health intervention for the management of anxiety and depression. *Int J Environ Res Public Health.* 2019;16(22):4413. doi:10.3390/ijerph16224413.

38 Rosa CD, Larson LR, Collado S, Profice CC. Forest therapy can prevent and treat depression: Evidence from meta-analyses. *Urban For Urban Green.* 2021;57:126943. doi:10.1016/j.ufug.2020.126943.

39 Whall AL, Black ME, Groh CJ, Yankou DJ, Kupferschmid BJ, Foster NL. The effect of natural environments upon agitation and aggression in late stage dementia patients. *Am J Alzheimers Dis.* 1997;12(5):216–220. doi:10.1177/153331759701200506.

40 Clark, Patrick, Mapes, Neil, Burt, Jim, Preston, Sarah. *Greening Dementia: A Literature Review of the Benefits and Barriers Facing Individuals Living with Dementia in Accessing the Natural Environment and Local Greenspace.* Natural England; 2013. http://publications.naturalengland.org.uk/publication/6578292471627776

41 Detweiler MB, Sharma T, Detweiler JG, et al. What is the evidence to support the use of therapeutic gardens for the elderly? *Psychiatry Investig.* 2012;9(2):100. doi:10.4306/pi.2012.9.2.100.

42 Mapes, Neil, Milton, Steve, Nicholls, Vicky, Williamson, Toby. *Is It Nice Outside? Consulting People Living with Dementia and Their Carers about Engaging with the Natural Environment.* Natural England; 2016. http://publications.naturalengland.org.uk/file/6209724725854208

43 Hewitt P, Watts C, Hussey J, Power K, Williams T. Does a structured gardening programme improve well-being in young-onset dementia? A preliminary study. *Br J Occup Ther.* 2013;76(8):355–361. doi:10.4276/030802213X13757040168270.

44 Healy V. The Hospice Garden: Addressing the patients' needs through landscape. *Am J Hosp Care.* 1986;3(6):32–36. doi:10.1177/104990918600300607.

45 Bell S de, White M, Griffiths A, et al. Spending time in the garden is positively associated with health and wellbeing: Results from a national survey in England. *Landsc Urban Plan.* 2020;200:103836. doi:10.1016/j.landurbplan.2020.103836.

46 Spano G, D'Este M, Giannico V, et al. Are community gardening and horticultural interventions beneficial for psychosocial well-being? A meta-analysis. *Int J Environ Res Public Health.* 2020;17(10):3584. doi:10.3390/ijerph17103584.

47 Porter R, McIlvaine-Newsad H. Gardening in green space for environmental justice: food security, leisure and social capital. *Leisure/Loisir.* 2013;37(4):379–395. doi:10.1080/14927713.2014.906172.

48 Parr H. *Mental Health and Social Space: Towards Inclusionary Geographies?* Blackwell; 2008.

49 Rayner M. The burden of food related ill health in the UK. *J Epidemiol Community Health.* 2005;59(12):1054–1057. doi:10.1136/jech.2005.036491.

50 Dauchet L, Amouyel P, Hercberg S, Dallongeville J. Fruit and vegetable consumption and risk of coronary heart disease: a meta-analysis of cohort studies. *J Nutr.* 2006;136(10):2588–2593. doi:10.1093/jn/136.10.2588.

51 Monlezun DJ, Kasprowicz E, Tosh KW, et al. Medical school-based teaching kitchen improves HbA1c, blood pressure, and cholesterol for patients with type 2 diabetes: results from a novel randomized controlled trial. *Diabetes Res Clin Pract.* 2015;109(2):420–426. doi:10.1016/j.diabres.2015.05.007.

52 Feinstein L, Hammond C, Woods L, University of London, Institute of Education, Centre for Research on the Wider Benefits of Learning. *The Contribution of Adult Learning to Health and Social Capital.* Institute of Education; 2003. https://discovery.ucl.ac.uk/id/eprint/10014854/1/WBLResRep8.pdf

53 u3a. University of the Third Age. https://www.u3a.org.uk/

54  Office for National Statistics. *National Life Tables – Life Expectancy in the UK: 2018 to 2020.* ONS; 2021. https://www.ons.gov.uk/peoplepopulationand community/birthsdeathsandmarriages/lifeexpectancies/bulletins/national lifetablesunitedkingdom/2018to2020

55  Office for National Statistics. *Suicides in England and Wales: 2020 Registrations.* ONS; 2021. https://www.ons.gov.uk/peoplepopulationandcommunity/birthsdeath sandmarriages/deaths/bulletins/suicidesintheunitedkingdom/2020registrations

56  Milligan C, Payne S, Bingley A, Cockshott Z. Place and wellbeing: shedding light on activity interventions for older men. *Ageing Soc.* 2015;35(1):124–149. doi:10.1017/S0144686X13000494.

57  Milligan C, Dowrick C. *Men in Sheds: Improving the Health and Wellbeing of Older Men through Gender-Based Activity Interventions: A Systematic Review and Scoping for an Evaluation.* School for Public Health Research; 2013. https://sphr. nihr.ac.uk/wp-content/uploads/2019/01/Men-in-Sheds-SPHR-Final-Report.pdf

58  Kelly D, Steiner A, Mason H, Teasdale S. Men's Sheds: A conceptual exploration of the causal pathways for health and well-being. *Health Soc Care Community.* 2019;27(5):1147–1157. doi:10.1111/hsc.12765.

59  Milligan C, Neary D, Payne S, Hanratty B, Irwin P, Dowrick C. Older men and social activity: a scoping review of Men's Sheds and other gendered interventions. *Ageing Soc.* 2016;36(5):895–923. doi:10.1017/S0144686X14001524.

60  Pit, Lianne. *An Explorative Research on the Reasons Why People Repair Their Product at the Repair Café.* Wageningen University; 2020. https://repaircafe.org/ wp-content/uploads/2020/05/Thesis_Lianne_Pit_februari_2020.pdf

61  Jarrott SE, Bruno K. Intergenerational activities involving persons with dementia: An observational assessment. *Am J Alzheimers Dis Other Demen.* 2003;18(1): 31–37. doi:10.1177/153331750301800109.

62  Eno, Brian. 2015 John Peel lecture. Delivered September 27, 2015. https://www. bbc.co.uk/mediacentre/speeches/2015/bbc-music-john-peel-lecture

63  Stendhal syndrome is named after the writer who had a transcendent experience on seeing frescoes in a Florentine church. Palacios-Sánchez L, Botero-Meneses JS, Pachón RP, Hernández LBP, Triana-Melo J del P, Ramírez-Rodríguez S. Stendhal syndrome: a clinical and historical overview. *Arq Neuropsiquiatr.* 2018;76(2):120–123. doi:10.1590/0004-282x20170189.

64  Angus J, University of Durham, Centre for Arts and Humanities in Health and Medicine, NHS Health Development Agency. *A Review of Evaluation in Community-Based Art for Health Activity in the UK.* Health Development Agency; 2002. https://www.artshealthresources.org.uk/wp-content/uploads/2017/01/2002-Angus-A-review-of-evaluation-in-community-arts-for-health-in-the-UK.pdf

65  Raw A, Lewis S, Russell A, Macnaughton J. A hole in the heart: confronting the drive for evidence-based impact research in arts and health. *Arts Health.* 2012;4(2):97–108. doi:10.1080/17533015.2011.619991.

66  Crone DM, O'Connell EE, Tyson PJ, Clark-Stone F, Opher S, James DVB. 'Art Lift' intervention to improve mental well-being: An observational study from UK general practice. *Int J Ment Health Nurs.* 2012;22(3):279–286. doi:10.1111/ j.1447-0349.2012.00862.x.

67  Hacking S, Secker J, Spandler H, Kent L, Shenton J. Evaluating the impact of participatory art projects for people with mental health needs. *Health Soc Care Community.* 2008;16(6):638–648. doi:10.1111/j.1365-2524.2008.00789.x.

68  Opher, Simon. *Cost-Benefit Evaluation of Artlift 2009-2012: Summary.* Artlift and NHS Gloucestershire; 2011. https://artlift.org/wp-content/uploads/2019/ 02/2009-2012-Simon-Opher-Cost-Benefit-Report.pdf

69  Venter E van de, Buller A. Arts on referral interventions: a mixed-methods study investigating factors associated with differential changes in mental well-being. *J Public Health.* 2014;37(1):143–150. doi:10.1093/pubmed/fdu028.

70 Frude N. Book prescriptions — a strategy for delivering psychological treatment in the primary care setting. *Ment Health Rev J*. 2005;10(4):30–33. doi:10.1108/13619322200500037.
71 Berthoud E, Elderkin S. *The Novel Cure: An A-Z of Literary Remedies*. Canongate; 2013.
72 The Reading Agency. Reading Well booklists for children. https://reading-well.org.uk/books/books-on-prescription/children
73 'Give sorrow words; the grief that does not speak knits up the o-er wrought heart and bids it break.' Macbeth, Act 4 Scene 3.
74 Unjudge someone. The Human Library Organization. https://humanlibrary.org/
75 Pennebaker JW, Seagal JD. Forming a story: the health benefits of narrative. *J Clin Psychol*. 1999;55(10):1243–1254.
76 Cohen GD, Perlstein S, Chapline J, Kelly J, Firth KM, Simmens S. The impact of professionally conducted cultural programs on the physical health, mental health, and social functioning of older adults—2-year results. *J Aging Humanit Arts*. 2007;1(1–2):5–22. doi:10.1080/19325610701410791.
77 Vella-Burrows T. *Singing and People with Dementia*. Sidney De Haan Centre for Arts and Health, Canterbury Christ Church University; 2012. https://www.artshealthresources.org.uk/docs/singing-and-people-with-dementia/
78 McNamara RJ, Epsley C, Coren E, McKeough ZJ. Singing for adults with chronic obstructive pulmonary disease. Cochrane Airways Group. *Cochrane Database Syst Rev*. 2017;2019(2). doi:10.1002/14651858.CD012296.pub2.
79 Clift S. *An Evaluation of Community Singing for People with COPD Chronic Obstructive Pulmonary Disease: Final Report*. Canterbury Christ Church University; 2013. https://www.canterbury.ac.uk/medicine-health-and-social-care/sidney-de-haan-research-centre/documents/research/Clift-Morrison-Skingley-Page-Coulton-Treadwell-VellaBurrows-Salisbury-Shipton-Evaluation-of-Community-Singing-for-People-with-COPD-FINAL.pdf
80 Morrison I, Clift, Stephen. *Singing and People with COPD (Chronic Obstructive Pulmonary Disease)*. Sidney De Haan Centre for Arts and Health, Canterbury Christ Church University; 2012. https://www.artshealthresources.org.uk/docs/singing-and-people-with-copd/
81 Antonovsky A. *Unraveling the Mystery of Health: How People Manage Stress and Stay Well*. Jossey-Bass; 1987.
82 Bandura A. Self-efficacy: toward a unifying theory of behavioral change. *Adv Behav Res Ther*. 1978;1(4):139–161. doi:10.1016/0146-6402(78)90002-4.
83 Maier SF, Seligman ME. Learned helplessness: theory and evidence. *J Exp Psychol Gen*. 1976;105(1):3–46. doi:10.1037/0096-3445.105.1.3.
84 Csikszentmihalyi M. *Flow and the Foundations of Positive Psychology*. Springer Netherlands; 2014. doi:10.1007/978-94-017-9088-8.

# 7    Social infrastructure

The richness and diversity of our communities is health-enabling, and developing associational life brings out the health benefits. Just as the best support for a tree is low down, allowing the stem to move, which encourages stronger roots, our social infrastructure is best nurtured rather than controlled. Support should be built in without being directive, feeding growth and enabling it to find its own space.

There is a risk of healthcare appropriating community assets to solve its own problems. Funding of healthcare services has a gravitational pull, sucking other provision into the realms of health. Commercial and political interests converge with a medicalised model that attributes illness to individual rather than systemic causes. Health services need to guard against this colonisation of community activity.

How do health and other statutory services support community development without being directive? It is the social infrastructure of our communities that generates connections and social capital. This is where support makes the most difference, nourishing without regulating.

Social infrastructure refers to the services and structures underlying associational life, the 'spaces that invite people into the public realm'.[1] Social infrastructure is shaped by the social norms that influence our interactions. Our physical 'hard' infrastructure can be designed to function as social infrastructure. These structures can be encouraged to be more health-generating, infrastructure designed to benefit health and wellbeing by default.

Our physical environment affects our social environment, which in turn influences our shared sense of cohesion as a community. The built and natural environments in which we live go as unremarked as the rests between musical notes. As we pass through these liminal spaces, we encounter and respond to people constantly, holding doors or changing our step to allow easier passing. Along with our more obvious associations, these micro-interactions in public spaces create our social environment. Small acts of courtesy promote and maintain social norms and sense of cohesion.

Every day, our lives bring a myriad of these interactions. There are people we regularly cross paths with who we may know only by sight. Recognition and awareness of the same people locally, known as a face-block community,[2] provides an important base level of sense of community which is

DOI: 10.4324/9781003391784-8

available to even the most isolated. Developing connections beyond mutual recognition needs a prompt to start, conversations often opening with a joke or an appraisal of the situation, perhaps because something out of the ordinary has happened. Sense of cohesion within a group also predisposes to conversation between group members.

Talking to others is good for us. Even just taking a moment to say thank you is linked to better wellbeing.[3] More purposeful spaces of group activity, known as micro-publics, bring people together, whether workplace, sports club or coffee shop. Transitory zones are the places we pass through during daily life.[4] These spaces provide plentiful opportunities for interactions, allowing cultural exchange and transformation.

Benches that encourage conversations are known as both listening and talking benches. Signs give permission for people to stop and talk: 'Happy to chat bench: sit here if you don't mind someone stopping to say hello'. These chance encounters have an impact that is far wider, enhancing our sense of coherence. Health Connections Mendip have taken this one step further, with a health connector visiting a bench weekly to be available to anyone who wants to talk.

Threshold spaces exist at the boundaries between private and communal space. These are spaces which offer the ability to experience associational life around us without having to join in. Front gardens and porches provide the opportunity for conversation if wished, or for just watching the world go by. Threshold spaces made prominent in the design of shared accommodation enable connections and provide distinctiveness, helping to maintain orientation.

Heritage forms an important part of place identification, giving local people an opportunity to shape how they see and present their community both to themselves and to visitors.[5] Residents choosing which aspects are worthy of conservation enhances local distinctiveness.

## Third places

Our public spaces can be laid out to promote socialisation. Community spaces open up opportunities for interactions, which increase social cohesion and capital. We spend most of our time in either our homes or workplaces, talking mainly with people already familiar to us. While these bonding conversations are crucial for our health, bridging connections with people we see less often are also important, both individually and societally. Spaces that allow wider interactions are known as *third places*,[6] forming the true heart of our communities, promoting contacts and encouraging interactions.

Third places are the stages for our associational lives, public squares, coffee shops, libraries and public houses offering space that is neither home nor work for serendipitous or planned meetings. A seat is really all that is needed to give permission to remain in a space, although shelter, toilets, a kettle and Wi-Fi increase the utility of that space greatly. Meetings outside of home or work avoid the obligations of guest or host, allowing people to join or leave when convenient. Even without conversing, third places provide vicarious companionship to those who are alone. Being around other people helps us feel connected. People watching lets us reflect on our social norms and understand the norms of those around us.

Being in a crowd or congregation increases our sense of cohesion. Festivals were originally disruptive events which temporarily subverted the usual hierarchies, but have become appropriated as spectacle, reinforcing corporate or state power, which has defused the radical ambition behind such events. Festivals that celebrate minority culture may actually reinforce the position of the majority as 'host'.[7]

Creating suitable spaces can be all that is needed to encourage interactions. The Camerados movement provides public living rooms (PLRs) as a space to chat and look out for each other.[8] PLRs can be based in public spaces or institutions like schools and hospitals. Camerados aim to be halfway between a stranger and a friend.[9] The ethos is not to try and fix someone, but to be alongside them, accepting that we can all be 'a bit rubbish sometimes'. Resisting the urge to find solutions enables different conversations, which find their own value.

Meeting places can be temporary, pop-up events such as community picnics or markets, or permanent, public spaces designed for interactions. Many town and village squares now provide outdoor, free-to-use gym equipment which encourages spending time in a shared environment. Third places need to be based in localities with safe walking access. The fundamentals are simple: a brew, a loo and something to do.[10]

Many third places are based around eating, drinking and chatting. Pubs are an important part of UK culture but are struggling, with six pubs closing every week.[11] Along with shops, community pubs can be retained as community assets by transferring ownership to local members, increasing connections and offering a wide range of services.[12] Parks and other outdoor venues are valuable third places, along with public services such as transport. Cemeteries are also public spaces that offer remembrance and reflection as well as biodiversity and greenspace. Libraries and other places open during the day allow us to be around others. This can be comforting for those with mental health issues, providing other voices which can distract from intrusive thoughts. Outdoor spaces and those with good ventilation have become especially important for those who need to minimise the risk of airborne infection.

## Greenspace

Ensuring our surroundings are sympathetic to nature improves wellbeing. Good design makes use of this to maximise the health and environmental benefits arising from connectedness with nature.

More than half the population of the world already lives in an urban environment, and by 2050 this is expected to have risen to two-thirds. The potential for health creation should be at the heart of urban design. The need for access to natural settings within urban environments is expressed in the *3-30-300 rule*.[13] This proposes that at least three trees should be visible from every home. Tree canopy cover should be at least thirty per cent, reducing pollution and noise exposure and encouraging time outdoors leading to interactions. The nearest greenspace should be accessible by a short walk of less than three hundred metres.

*Table 7.1* Value of greenspace

| | |
|---|---|
| Parks | The return on investment is £34 for every £1 spent on parks, due to increased physical activity, better mental health, carbon storage, improved air quality and reduced crime.[a] £111 mn is saved in reduced GP visits, and £34 bn overall wellbeing benefit from frequent use of parks and greenspace.[b] |
| Access | Minimum guidance is that everyone should have at least two hectares (200 m × 100 m) of natural greenspace within 500 m of their home, and at least one 100 hectare (1,000 m × 1,000 m) site within 5 km.[c] |
| 3-30-300 rule | 3 trees visible from every home, 30% tree canopy coverage (canopy coverage in London is 21%), 300 m maximum to nearest greenspace.[d] |
| Trees | 8.4 mn trees in London bring £132 mn benefit annually, by removing pollution, storing carbon, slowing stormwater and reducing building energy costs.[e] Greater vegetation cover is associated with a lower risk of schizophrenia[f] and dementia.[g] Trees slow driving speeds and reduce crime rates.[h] Street trees save £16 mn a year in antidepressant costs.[i] |

Notes:
a Eis, Jason. The economics of urban parks. Presented at: Prosperous Cities Conference; September 27, 2016; London. https://www.vivideconomics.com/wp-content/uploads/2019/08/Prosperous-cities-conference-slides.pdf
b Fields in Trust. *Revaluing Parks and Green Spaces: Measuring Their Economic and Wellbeing Value to Individuals*; 2018. https://www.fieldsintrust.org/revaluing
c Box, John, Harrison, Carolyn. Natural spaces in urban places. *Town Ctry Plan.* 1993; 62(9):231–235.
d Konijnendijk van den Bosch, Cecil. The 3-30-300 rule for urban forestry and greener cities. *Biophilic Cities J.* 2021;4(2). https://www.researchgate.net/publication/353571108_The_3-30-300_Rule_for_Urban_Forestry_and_Greener_Cities
e Rogers K, Sacre K, Goodenough J, Doick KJ. *Valuing London's Urban Forest: Results of the London i-Tree Eco Project*. Treeconomics; 2015. https://www.london.gov.uk/sites/default/files/valuing_londons_urban_forest_i-tree_report_final.pdf
f Engemann K, Pedersen CB, Arge L, Tsirogiannis C, Mortensen PB, Svenning JC. Childhood exposure to green space – A novel risk-decreasing mechanism for schizophrenia? *Schizophr Res.* 2018;199:142–148. doi:10.1016/j.schres.2018.03.026.
g Mmako NJ, Courtney-Pratt H, Marsh P. Green spaces, dementia and a meaningful life in the community: a mixed studies review. *Health Place.* 2020;63:102344. doi:10.1016/j.healthplace.2020.102344.
h Hastie, Chris. *The Benefits of Urban Trees*. Warwick District Council; 2003. https://www.naturewithin.info/UF/TreeBenefitsUK.pdf
i Saraev, Vadim, O'Brien, Liz, Valatin, Gregory, Bursnell, Matthew. *Valuing the Mental Health Benefits of Woodlands*. Forest Research; 2021. https://cdn.forestresearch.gov.uk/2021/12/frrp034.pdf

Parks provide the most convenient access to greenspace for many people, with almost half of adults in England visiting a park at least weekly.[14] The cost-benefits parks bring to the local population are substantial but invisible, as the financial return is hidden within expensive health care that was not needed. Parks save healthcare costs and reduce disparities, the shared space for play and meeting others particularly important to people who are marginalised. An uplift in local house prices also contributes to the increase in value, though this brings a risk that greening urban areas displaces lower-income households, paradoxically worsening inequality. Promotional events, good active transport links, lower traffic speeds and diverse land use all encourage activity, generating greenspace benefits.[15]

Trees and greenspace promote social cohesion and help place identification. One in ten trees in inner London are fruit trees, providing biodiversity and food for humans and wildlife alike. Trees make homes more desirable, improving air quality, reducing energy costs and providing shading and attenuation of storm water. Street trees help cool urban spaces by creating a cooling microclimate. Antidepressant prescriptions fall for every extra street tree per kilometre, even after adjusting for variables such as income and deprivation.[16] The value to humans that trees bring was demonstrated by a noticeable increase in human deaths after the emerald ash borer pest spread across the United States, killing tens of millions of ash trees. Deaths from cardiovascular and respiratory conditions increased in affected states.[17]

Trees are the largest manifestation of nature in urban environments, but at ground level dandelions and weeds provide food for pollinators, and saplings of pioneer species scramble up through gaps in car parks and pavements. Nature is all around us, when we look.

## Dementia friendly communities

Ensuring our publicly accessible spaces are inclusive considers the specific needs of people with sensory and cognitive issues, who tend to be overlooked in the design of our towns and cities and the way our lives are organised. Similar principles apply when creating environments suitable for people with physical disabilities and with sensory problems such as those associated with autism. People with dementia benefit from walking, which gives purpose and preserves fitness. Slopes are safer than steps at reducing falls, while buffer zones protect walkways from traffic. Greenspace, good lighting, accessible toilets and seating which does not conduct heat or cold all invite journeys by foot.

Although walking is usually purposeful, being found 'wandering' strongly predicts entering residential care. Distractions such as noise or roadworks can temporarily disorientate, leading to getting lost. Good urban layout helps orientation, forks and T-junctions being easier to navigate than crossroads. Streets that meander and contain interesting or memorable landmarks improve orientation. Exposure to natural light and greenery helps maintain awareness of time and season, and reduces evening agitation, known as sundowning.[18]

Spaces such as wander gardens for people with dementia provide circular walks with no dead ends. Planting should aim to stimulate all five senses, using non-toxic plants chosen for sound, texture and scent and shaded seating suitable for group activities. Raised beds enable wheelchair accessible gardening, needing paths wide enough for two wheelchairs to pass. Changes in flooring colour should be avoided as a sudden darker shade can be perceived as a hole, while using low-glare surfaces reduces the impact of visual problems. Curiosity about how the next view will open up encourages progress through the garden.

Dementia friendly communities provide infrastructure that is familiar, legible, distinctive, accessible, comfortable and safe.[19] Local shops in particular can support people with dementia to remain independent. Shops are important third places which help to anchor communities and provide strong place identification. Good shop design improves accessibility, with consistent logos and signage helpful for people who are reliant on visual cues for location. Signs need to be clear and notable but not cluttered, with consistent, contrasting colours. Using warmer colour hues of reds and oranges reduces the impact of colour agnosia, which makes blues and greens harder to distinguish. Staff in shops and businesses should be able to access an ongoing program of dementia friends training, which raises awareness and tackles misconceptions around dementia.

The design of much of the residential estate for older people is not conducive to interactions. Without suitable shared spaces, elderly people become trapped behind their front doors. Better access to public transport reduces the impacts of inequality and keeps people mobile and more economically active into older years, as well as providing an important third place for connections and chance encounters.

---

**Box 7.1   Dementia meeting centre**

Ross Meeting Centre opened in 2017. This is for people with mild to moderate dementia and their carers, meeting weekly for lunch, activities and fun. The meeting centre model originated in the Netherlands. What makes it work is the involvement of carers and volunteers, who share in the activities. Spending time with other carers builds support networks, sharing information and modelling behaviours. This shared knowledge forms a powerful community health asset. Attending meeting centres reduces carer strain and delays institutionalisation.[20]

---

## Road infrastructure

City streets used to be considered public spaces, but increasing numbers of traffic casualties led the automobile lobby to divert accountability by promoting the idea that streets are for vehicles. The pejorative term 'jaywalker' was used in the US to describe pedestrians crossing streets, Boy Scouts handing out cards informing people of the risks of jaywalking in the name of safety.[21] This normalised travelling at speed through populated areas and transferred blame for collisions onto vulnerable road users such as pedestrians and cyclists.

Language used in reports of crashes continues to betray a bias towards victim blaming. Describing cars rather than drivers crashing acts to shift culpability away from drivers.[22] Calling vehicle crashes 'accidents' minimises the dangers inherent in our current transport policy. The dominance of vehicles in our culture is rarely questioned.

Cyclists, motorcyclists and pedestrians have the highest mortality per mile travelled.[23] Child pedestrian casualty rates in the UK are among the worst in Europe, but this would be easy to improve; 20 mph zones reduce death and injury by 40 per cent.[24] A vehicle travelling at 30 mph transfers more than twice as much energy in a collision as one travelling at 20 mph. Addressing this avoidable and tragic loss of life means recognising how vehicle-centric design has made our transport system so dangerous to others.

Transport choices impact on physical activity, air pollution and the local environment. Road traffic casualties are the most obvious health impact of transport, but pollution by particulates and greenhouse gases causes invisible but even greater health-limiting effects. Premature deaths due to air pollution from the combustion engine outnumber road deaths by fifteen to one. Electric vehicles avoid tailpipe pollution from combustion but still produce particulate air pollution from tyres and brakes.

The UK government spends only 1 per cent of the £27 bn road budget on active travel, instead heavily subsidising transport modalities which are damaging to our health. Repairing roads is a huge cost burden for local authorities, coming from a budget ultimately shared with education and social care. The increasing size of cars not only restricts visibility of vulnerable road users, especially children, but wastes money on road repairs, as damage to roads increases exponentially with weight. [25] Every car journey replaced saves money for councils.

Splay of roads at junctions encourages speed and makes crossing longer and more dangerous. The tracks vehicles leave when it snows show how much road space is wasted, space that could have communal use. Pedestrianising streets reclaims these spaces, increasing employment and trade in local shops as well as benefiting health.[26]

Most cities are still dominated by cars and roads, making active travel choices such as walking less inviting, which contributes to obesity and cardiovascular risk. This recognition has led to the 'fifteen-minute city' concept, whereby essential services are available to all within fifteen minutes by foot or safe cycle route. Primary services such as shops and transport hubs should be within five hundred metres of homes, and secondary services such as health centres and places of worship within eight hundred metres.[27] Reducing car use means prioritising safe cycling and walking infrastructure, combined with public transport so good that even the wealthy use it.[28]

Four times as many people walk when pavements are suitable and safe.[29] Low traffic neighbourhoods (LTNs) preferentially allow pedestrian and cycle access via modal filters which restrict motor vehicles. LTNs reduce car use, traffic noise and speed and increase walking and cycling in residents by more than two hours a week,[30] as well as lowering street crime and injuries from road traffic collisions.[31] The reduction in air pollution from LTNs is enough to improve average life expectancy by around six weeks.[32]

Showing the effects of pollution sends a powerful health message on this avoidable cause of death. Leaving combustion engines idling when not moving contributes significantly to air pollution. Clean Air Zones can be

*Table 7.2* Health impacts of traffic

| | |
|---|---|
| Road deaths | There were 1,752 road deaths in Britain in 2019, each losing an average of 35 life years.[a] |
| Vehicle speed | The risk of pedestrian injury or death increases significantly with speed:<br>• 5% at 20 mph<br>• 45% at 30 mph<br>• 85% at 40 mph |
| 20mph zones | 1,000 casualties are prevented annually in London by 20 mph zones. 700 further casualties would be prevented by rolling out 20 mph zones across London.[b] |
| LTNs | Low traffic neighbourhoods lead to a 75% reduction in road traffic injuries.[c] |
| Cars | Roads and vehicles take up large areas of civic space, parked cars in London taking up 14 km² (2%) of land. |
| Roads | The budget for new roads would instead fund a thousand new parks, saving 74,000 tonnes of $CO_2$ each year.[d] |
| Bus journeys | Improving bus services reduces local deprivation with a wider ROI of 3.62.[e] |
| Air quality | Poor air quality in the UK, predominantly due to traffic emissions, causes 29,000 early deaths each year losing 340,000 years of life, costing up to 3.5% of GDP.[f] |

Notes:
a Department for Transport. Reported road casualties Great Britain, provisional results: 2020. National statistics. Published June 24, 2021. https://www.gov.uk/government/statistics/reported-road-casualties-great-britain-provisional-results-2020/reported-road-casualties-great-britain-provisional-results-2020
b Grundy, Chris, Steinbach, Rebecca, Edwards, Phil, Wilkinson, Paul, Green, Judith. *The Effect of 20mph Zones on Inequalities in Road Casualties in London: A Report to the London Road Safety Unit.* London School of Hygiene and Tropical Medicine; 2008. https://content.tfl.gov.uk/the-effect-of-20-mph-zones-on-inequalities-in-road-casualties-in-london.pdf
c Laverty AA, Goodman A, Aldred R. Low traffic neighbourhoods and population health. *BMJ*. 2021;372. doi:10.1136/bmj.n443.
d Marmot, Michael, Allen, Jessica, Goldblatt, Peter, et al. *Fair Society, Healthy Lives: The Marmot Review.* UCL; 2010.
e A 10% improvement in local bus connections is associated with a 3.6% reduction in deprivation (IMD). KPMG. *A Study of the Value of Local Bus Services to Society: A Report for Greener Journeys.* University of Leeds; 2016. https://www.cpt-uk.org/media/yqsda4iu/greener-journeys-value-of-bus-to-society-final-1.pdf
f Yim SHL, Barrett SRH. Public health impacts of combustion emissions in the United Kingdom. *Environ Sci Technol.* 2012;46(8):4291–4296. doi:10.1021/es2040416.

instituted by local authorities, either chargeable or advisory.[33] Especially around schools and health facilities, these help to emphasise the damage caused by air pollution.

Last mile delivery schemes avoid the most costly and the most polluting last mile of delivery. Walkable collection points reduce emissions and encourage activity and interactions. Electric cargo bikes have the potential to revolutionise last mile services, lowering emissions in more populated areas.

## Active by design

Better access to physical activity through our lives is crucial to our health, and even small increases in exertion are very beneficial. Building activity by default into our infrastructure improves health outcomes, helping to counter the differences in mortality caused by inequality. Health-by-design approaches promote healthy options by making walking and taking the stairs more convenient than taking the car or escalator. Walking is therapeutic for people with vascular problems, as it maintains the arterial blood supply to the legs, reducing the risk of needing surgery. Ample provision of seating makes walking more feasible for the elderly and those with limited mobility.

Active travel is the best way to integrate activity into daily life. The activity from cycling, for instance, prevents over two thousand premature deaths in the UK annually. The perception that a certain level of fitness is required is no longer true, as electric bikes have increased the range and lowered the effort necessary, making a bicycle feasible for far more journeys. Cargo bikes increase carrying capacity, including the ability to transport children.

Overwhelmingly the biggest risk factor to cyclists is motor vehicles, but the road safety debate has instead focused on the use of cycle helmets and whether these should be mandatory. The suggestion that better safety wear is needed to prevent injury to cyclists shifts blame towards the victim and away from the need for better infrastructure. There is evidence of risk compensation by drivers who pass nearer to cyclists wearing helmets.[34] Mandating helmets reduces cycling, such that the lives lost from the reduction in exercise more than outweigh any reduction in head injury. Making helmets compulsory would lead to up to eight hundred extra deaths each year in the UK.[35]

Embracing active travel has benefits for both climate and the local environment. Weaning ourselves from our reliance on vehicles and shifting to low-carbon modes of transport reduces the burden on our environment, improving air quality and fitness. Temporarily closing streets to motor vehicles, known as open streets,[36] or Ciclovía, is a useful way to improve confidence and support active transport in a safe and fun environment. The most effective way to encourage modal transport shift longer term is to build safe active travel infrastructure. Cycle lanes should be physically protected from traffic, as the risk of collision is actually increased in advisory lanes that vehicles are allowed to enter.[37] Safe cycle lanes and facilities to lock bikes open up cycling to wider participation.

## Community engagement

Place-based interventions to improve health are within the gift of communities, but understanding what works and putting it in place is an ongoing, iterative process. Much of the responsibility for infrastructure lies with local councils, which should reflect the views of citizens, who in turn need to be able to hold councils to account. Developing social infrastructure needs meaningful engagement and participation from citizens. Empowered residents are able to make changes, influencing the attitudes of others when shown change is possible.

There are four main strands to developing the health aspects of our communities:[38]

* Building community capacity
* Building individual capabilities
* Improving collaboration
* Connecting to community resources

These strands overlap and interweave to achieve empowerment, equity and social connectedness. Enhancing volunteering and peer support improves individual capabilities. Strengthening the capacity of communities to take action on health allows the identification of local issues and sharing of solutions. An infrastructure of community connectors is an effective way to promote engagement. Resources such as library hubs support and link people and organisations. The common factor is the investment of the local community in ensuring progress.

Community engagement ensures involvement in decisions on everything from design, procurement, delivery and governance.[39] Feedback from a representative group of citizens is invaluable but can be hard to access. While online engagement is a cheap and convenient way to reach people, using this alone reinforces the digital divide. Social media is still often viewed as a one-way method of propagating information, rather than a true opportunity for dialogue.[40]

*Table 7.3* Community engagement[a]

| Community-oriented | Doing to | The community is informed |
|---|---|---|
| Community-based | Doing for | Consultation and involvement of the community |
| Community-managed | Doing with | Collaboration with community leaders |
| Community-owned | Doing by | Empowerment of the community to develop systems and assets |

Note:
a World Health Organization. *Community Engagement: A Health Promotion Guide for Universal Health Coverage in the Hands of the People.* World Health Organization; 2020. https://apps.who.int/iris/handle/10665/334379

Trust, accessibility, context, equity, transparency and autonomy are important principles of community engagement.[41] These factors interact; trust needs transparency, while improving access for marginalised groups increases equity. Leadership, communication and shared decision-making are necessary for change to happen.

Involving communities in research ensures local priorities are respected. Rather than the traditional focus on counting what is quantifiable, participatory action research (PAR) is a bottom-up approach looking at community empowerment.[42] The aim is to reach and include marginalised groups and reduce health inequalities.[43]

Improving information flow, promoting community governance and developing social capital all help to develop empowered communities and improve the health of participants. Barriers include lack of community capacity, lack of engagement, cultural constraints, transaction costs and the misuse of professional power. A lack of coherency within government planning and a centrally driven focus on quick wins has distracted from attempts at true community engagement.[44]

*Table 7.4* Evidence for community initiatives[a]

| | | *Strength of evidence* |
|---|---|---|
| Economic outcomes | Employment, directly within community infrastructure or by increasing skills and encouraging new business | + |
| | Higher social capital adds economic value | ++ |
| Health outcomes | Reduced mortality and improved quality of life due to social networks | ++ |
| | Better mental health and lower health-care usage | ++ |
| | Health-enabling behaviour | + |
| Social outcomes | Networks provide resilience | +++ |
| | Wellbeing through public spaces, greenspace, connectedness and volunteering | ++++ |
| | Less loneliness, increased opportunities for interactions | + |
| | Reductions in crime | + |
| Civic outcomes | Social cohesion | ++ |
| | Social inclusion | + |
| | Stronger sense of belonging, ownership and pride | ++ |

Notes:
a World Health Organization. *Community Engagement: A Health Promotion Guide for Universal Health Coverage in the Hands of the People.* World Health Organization; 2020. https://apps.who.int/iris/handle/10665/334379

(Strength of evidence: very strong ++++, strong +++, medium ++, limited +)

Accepting ownership by communities can feel difficult for statutory services who are used to having control and may be hesitant to cede this. The purpose is to give better local control of priorities in order to have ownership of the outcomes and share in the solutions.

There is a danger that community assets may be used to replace existing services, fulfilling an organisational rather than community agenda. Market-driven 'asset stripping' in this way maximises short term profits but externalises responsibilities. Development from the ground up, by an empowered community, builds more adaptive and responsive structures.

Service, working with individuals, and advocacy, working on behalf of others, both improve lives but usually fail to challenge or improve relationships with institutions. It is mobilisation that builds power.[45] Mobilising is considered a short-term response, but one that can lead to organising, which is a more effective way to arrange ongoing efforts without having to rebuild structures each time. Organisations bring efficiencies and skills, although this requires longer-term thinking than single-issue campaigning needs.

### Ensuring true participation

There is a spectrum of engagement, building up to true citizen power (Table 7.5). The dominance of power structures underlying a hierarchical society means that most attempts at community engagement end up reinforcing the status quo.[46] At the lowest level of involvement, the needs of citizens are invoked purely to support the needs of the organisation. Groups are gathered by those in power in order to demonstrate legitimacy, providing participation in name only. Without any redistribution of power, participation is empty, but allows system architects to maintain the illusion of engagement.

*Table 7.5*  Degrees of participation, (Sherry Arnstein)[a]

| Degrees of citizen power | Citizen control | True community governance |
|---|---|---|
| | Delegated power | Citizens become dominant |
| | Partnership | Citizens are legitimate stakeholders, sharing decisions through negotiation |
| Degrees of tokenism | Placation | Token appointments to boards or advisory committees |
| | Consultation | Feedback |
| | Informing | The start of a dialogue, but one that is one-way |
| Nonparticipation | Therapy | Policy aims to educate or cure citizens |
| | Manipulation | Citizens used to lend legitimacy to plans |

Note:
a Arnstein SR. A ladder of citizen participation. *J Am Inst Plann.* 1969;35(4):216–224. doi:10.1080/01944366908977225.

The state may see citizens as being in need of 'cure'. Social iatrogenesis pathologises citizens, justifying external intervention and control. A deficit-based model of communities hides oppression under the cover of creating a model society. As engagement grows, contributions from the community may be considered, but the power to make decisions remains elsewhere. Attempts at communication need to be two-way, but are meaningless until they lead to influence.

As community voices start being heard, representative participation starts to reduce dependency and rebalance the power within relationships. True engagement begins when partnership is shared with citizens, transformative participation ensuring decisions are community based and enacted.[47] Ultimately, institutions have to get out of the way for true citizen control.

## Power

Power is the capacity to influence. Both individuals and groups can hold power, and power can be over ourselves as well as over others. Enhancing ways to control our own lives is known as *empowerment*. Power can be zerosum, where it can only change hands, or not zero-sum, where resources can increase over time. Within the ideology of capitalism, power can only be gained if it is lost somewhere else, explaining why those in control are resistant to sharing power.

The idea that value comes only from scarcity misses the symbiotic gains from working together. Power that is not zero-sum is not only possible but widespread; a parent, teacher or mentor gains directly and indirectly from teaching skills to others. The benefits of volunteering to those who volunteer are ample demonstration of how helping others helps oneself. This positive-sum process becomes self-reinforcing, increasing power within the community as well as within individuals. This 'synergy' paradigm presents an alternative to the 'scarcity' model, recognising that human resources are renewable and expandable.[48] In the virtuous circle of social capital, empowerment benefits all, trust engendering trust, transforming time invested into improved relationships. Adding to the liberation of another enhances one's own power.

*Table 7.6* Types of power[a]

| | |
|---|---|
| Reward | Power reinforced by rewards |
| Coercive | Power enforced by negative consequences for nonconformity |
| Legitimate | Structurally conferred power |
| Expert | Power derived from superior knowledge |
| Informational | Data which can influence or persuade a course of action |
| Referent | Influence through respect or admiration, recognisable within healthcare as transference |

Note:
a French JRP, Raven B. The bases of social power. In: Cartwright D, ed. *Studies in Social Power*; 1959:150–167.

'Power-over' is the most familiar form of power, in which one party acts at the will of another, even when it may not be in their best interests. This is dominant where it is enforced by threats, hegemonic if using persuasion or exploitation, or indirect, typically via economic control which causes inequalities to persist.[49] Structural violence, when damage is caused by the denial of basic needs, is built on dominant power structures. Hegemonic power is most commonly used by professionals, asserting an expert view which risks overriding the concerns of the individual.

## Powerlessness

'Power-within' is an expression of self, of gaining control over one's situation. Powerlessness is the opposite, where outcomes are outside one's control. Internalising existing power structures leads to helplessness and powerlessness. Lack of control, whether in the workplace or as a result of a dispute, is a very common precursor in clinical practice to a presentation with depression.

Not everyone wants to be empowered. Oppression, whether overt or subtle, can persuade people that they do not have the right to power. Internalising blame diminishes our sense of self, and normalises the idea that others could and should play the lead role in our stories. This takeover of our narratives discourages the possibility of a change of control, instead shaping us into passive consumers, decisions taken on our behalf. When fear of failure stops us from trying, or when consistent failure to change things leads to apathy and learned helplessness, powerlessness becomes compounded by the belief that the situation is immutable. Oppression comes from the burden of change being put on the individual, which avoids the need for systemic change.

The prevailing narrative within our society is of success through one's efforts, which reinforces the effects of perceived failure by the standards of this social norm. We are told that we are responsible for our happiness, our successes and our failures, driving feelings of worthlessness against ideals of perfection against which we are all found wanting. The ideology of neoliberalism promotes individualism and competition, but shows little regard for others along the way.

Vast economic power is concentrated in the hands of a few, who use this to maintain political power. This framework is accepted uncritically by people and institutions, reinforced by the fear that things would be worse if the status quo were not maintained. This is real powerlessness, which becomes *surplus powerlessness* when the belief that things cannot change becomes pervasive.[50]

There are some similarities between powerlessness and *impostor phenomenon* (also known as impostor syndrome, although conceptualising this as a syndrome inappropriately pathologises these common feelings). Those seeing themselves as impostors feel unable and unworthy, despite evidence to the contrary. This self-deception may be a feature of those lacking support in childhood,[51] especially where qualities are seen as being fixed rather than mutable. Internalising beliefs that failure is due to personal deficiencies makes it harder to believe in one's own power.

Choice, whether in the voting booth or supermarket, is a helpful proxy for power. In both of these situations, there are complex forces striving to influence our behaviour, including using the various datasets about us to predict and steer us most effectively. We lose power whenever our behaviour is modulated by others. In this case, power is zero-sum; what we lose, someone else gains.

## Empowerment

The promise of power is often used to tempt us. The political slogan 'take back control' effectively played into widespread feelings of powerlessness, externalising blame for the effects of austerity and promising an increase in 'power-within' while deftly reinforcing the status quo. Deliberately empowering another is problematic, more akin to rescuing than sharing. Power cannot be given, only taken. Creating the conditions to allow people to discover their own power is sufficient. Recognising our own needs and motives is necessary to engage with others meaningfully: 'If you come because your liberation is bound up in mine, then let us begin'.[52]

'Power-over' can be used to nurture 'power-within', as the locus of control becomes internalised. This is the basis of much of the therapeutic relationship, but the same dynamic occurs at community scale. Identifying sources of power-within is necessary to facilitate a therapeutic transfer of power. There are parallels with transactional analysis, as relationships shift from parent-child to adult-adult.[53] Recognising strengths provides stable foundations on which to expand repertoires and build confidence. Identifying assets in this way is as important for individuals as it is for communities. Respecting priorities avoids inadvertent hegemonic control and maximises the sense of 'power-within'.

## Activism

Activism can be a form of sublimation, a psychological defence mechanism which finds a healthy way to channel distress into a productive process. Changing the world entails changing ourselves.

Individual empowerment begins when our sense of integrity is violated.[54] We all have different thresholds and triggers for this happening, so we each start the journey alone. There are similarities with coming of age and maturing as an individual, just as our relationship with our parents or carers changes over time. Recognising that those with power are not qualitatively different to us expands our possible relationships to authority. Just as we grow from child to adult to parent, our sense of agency comes from recognising our choice over which role to play.

If sudden individual empowerment is an epiphany, it still takes the support of others to consolidate this position. Peer discussion helps the development of critical structural understanding. Mentoring relationships encourage progress through reflection. Resistance will inevitably be encountered along the way, as autocratic systems try to reject attempts at subversion. External support helps frame these conflicts within a wider context to encourage perseverance.

'Incorporation' describes the maturation of the political self, when impediments are recognised and the landscape understood. Activism and leadership become entwined, although identifying as a leader can be uncomfortable for those who reject traditional hierarchies. Ongoing conflict is challenging, but critical to making change. The final stage, commitment, recognises that activism is possible across a wide range of endeavours; it matters less exactly where we put our shoulders to the wheel.

## Notes

Links and additional resources for this chapter can be found at www.communityhealth.uk/7-social-infrastructure

1 Klinenberg E. *Palaces for the People: How to Build a More Equal and United Society*. Penguin Random House; 2020.
2 Suttles GD. *The Social Construction of Communities*. Univ. of Chicago Press; 1973.
3 Gunaydin G, Oztekin H, Karabulut DH, Salman-Engin S. Minimal social interactions with strangers predict greater subjective well-being. *J Happiness Stud.* 2021;22(4):1839–1853. doi:10.1007/s10902-020-00298-6.
4 Yarker S. *Creating Spaces for an Ageing Society: The Role of Critical Social Infrastructure*. Emerald Publishing; 2022.
5 Alexander M, Hamilton K. Recapturing place identification through community heritage marketing. *Eur J Mark.* 2016;50(7/8):1118–1136. doi:10.1108/EJM-05-2013-0235.
6 Oldenburg R, Brissett D. The third place. *Qual Sociol.* 1982;5(4):265–284. doi:10.1007/BF00986754.
7 Fincher R, Iveson K. *Planning and Diversity in the City: Redistribution, Recognition and Encounter*. Palgrave Macmillan; 2008.
8 Camerados. Get through and get each other through tough times. https://www.camerados.org/
9 Batty, Elaine, Bennett, Ellen, Devany, Chris, Harris, Cathy, Pearson, Sarah, Woodward, Abi. *Friends and Purpose: Evaluation of Camerados Public Living Rooms*. Sheffield Hallam University Centre for Regional Economic and Social Research; 2020. https://shura.shu.ac.uk/26043/
10 Jones, Dan, Jopling, Kate, Kharicha, Kalpa. *Loneliness beyond Covid-19: Learning the Lessons of the Pandemic for a Less Lonely Future*. Campaign to End Loneliness; 2021. https://www.campaigntoendloneliness.org/wp-content/uploads/Loneliness-beyond-Covid-19-July-2021.pdf
11 Campaign for Real Ale. *Pub Closure Report 2021*. CAMRA; 2022. https://camra.org.uk/campaign_resources/camra-pub-closure-report-2021/
12 Plunkett Foundation. *Community Pubs: A Better Form of Business*; 2020. https://plunkett.co.uk/community-owned-pubs-and-shops-show-resilience-in-the-face-of-covid-19/
13 Konijnendijk van den Bosch, Cecil. The 3-30-300 rule for urban forestry and greener cities. *Biophilic Cities J.* 2021;4(2). https://www.researchgate.net/publication/353571108_The_3-30-300_Rule_for_Urban_Forestry_and_Greener_Cities
14 Kaźmierczak A. The contribution of local parks to neighbourhood social ties. *Landsc Urban Plan.* 2013;109(1):31–44. doi:10.1016/j.landurbplan.2012.05.007.
15 Sallis JF, Spoon C, Cavill N, et al. Co-benefits of designing communities for active living: an exploration of literature. *Int J Behav Nutr Phys Act.* 2015;12(1):30. doi:10.1186/s12966-015-0188-2.

16  Taylor MS, Wheeler BW, White MP, Economou T, Osborne NJ. Research note: Urban street tree density and antidepressant prescription rates – A cross-sectional study in London, UK. *Landsc Urban Plan.* 2015;136:174–179. doi:10.1016/j. landurbplan.2014.12.005.

17  Mortality from cardiovascular and respiratory conditions in affected states rose by 23 extra deaths annually per 100,000 adults. Donovan GH, Butry DT, Michael YL, et al. The relationship between trees and human health. *Am J Prev Med.* 2013;44(2):139–145. doi:10.1016/j.amepre.2012.09.066.

18  Mitchell L, Burton E. Designing dementia-friendly neighbourhoods: helping people with dementia to get out and about. *J Integr Care.* 2010;18(6):11–18. doi:10.5042/jic.2010.0647.

19  Mitchell L, Burton E. Neighbourhoods for life: Designing dementia-friendly outdoor environments. *Qual Ageing Older Adults.* 2006;7(1):26–33. doi:10.1108/ 14717794200600005.

20  Dröes RM, Breebaart E, Meiland FJM, van Tilburg W, Mellenbergh GJ. Effect of meeting centres support program on feelings of competence of family carers and delay of institutionalization of people with dementia. *Aging Ment Health.* 2004;8(3):201–211. doi:10.1080/13607860410001669732.

21  Norton PD. *Fighting Traffic: The Dawn of the Motor Age in the American City.* MIT Press; 2008.

22  Ralph K, Iacobucci E, Thigpen CG, Goddard T. Editorial patterns in bicyclist and pedestrian crash reporting. *Transp Res Rec J Transp Res Board.* 2019;2673(2):663–671. doi:10.1177/0361198119825637.

23  Department for Transport. Reported road casualties Great Britain, provisional results: 2020. National statistics. Published June 24, 2021. https://www.gov.uk/ government/statistics/reported-road-casualties-great-britain-provisional- results-2020/reported-road-casualties-great-britain-provisional-results-2020

24  Marmot, Michael, Allen, Jessica, Goldblatt, Peter, et al. *Fair Society, Healthy Lives: The Marmot Review.* UCL; 2010. https://www.instituteofhealthequity.org/ resources-reports/fair-society-healthy-lives-the-marmot-review

25  Road damage is related to the fourth power of vehicle weight, meaning the damage to road surfaces from a car is 160,000 times that of a bicycle, and a lorry the same again compared to a car. Yiu, Yuen. How much damage do heavy trucks do to our roads? Inside Science. Published October 12, 2020. https://insidescience. org/news/how-much-damage-do-heavy-trucks-do-our-roads

26  Soni N, Soni N. Benefits of pedestrianization and warrants to pedestrianize an area. *Land Use Policy.* 2016;57:139–150. doi:10.1016/j.landusepol.2016.05.009.

27  See note 18.

28  Peñalosa, Enrique. Why buses represent democracy in action. September 2013. https://www.youtube.com/watch?v=j3YjeARuilI

29  Jacobsen PL, Racioppi F, Rutter H. Who owns the roads? How motorised traffic discourages walking and bicycling. *Inj Prev.* 2009;15(6):369–373. doi:10.1136/ ip.2009.022566.

30  Aldred R, Goodman A. Low Traffic Neighbourhoods, car use, and active travel: evidence from the people and places survey of Outer London active travel interventions. *Findings.* Published online September 2020. doi:10.32866/001c.17128.

31  Laverty AA, Goodman A, Aldred R. Low traffic neighbourhoods and population health. *BMJ.* 2021;372. doi:10.1136/bmj.n443.

32  Dajnak D, Walton H, Stewart G, Smith JD, Beevers S. *Air Quality: Concentrations, Exposure and Attitudes in Waltham Forest.* Kings College London; 2018. https:// www.cycling-embassy.org.uk/sites/cycling-embassy.org.uk/files/documents/ WalthamForest_Kings%20Report_310718.pdf

33  Department for Environment Food and Rural Affairs, Department for Transport. *Clean Air Zone Framework: Principles for Setting up Clean Air Zones in England.* UK Government; 2020. https://www.gov.uk/government/publications/air-quality- clean-air-zone-framework-for-england

34 Walker I. Drivers overtaking bicyclists: objective data on the effects of riding position, helmet use, vehicle type and apparent gender. *Accid Anal Prev.* 2007;39(2):417–425. doi:10.1016/j.aap.2006.08.010.

35 Gleave, James. *Cycle Helmets: The Impacts of Compulsory Cycle Helmet Legislation on Cyclist Fatalities and Premature Deaths in the UK.* Transport Planning Society; 2012:25. http://www.cycle-helmets.com/helmets-uk-dec-2012. pdf

36 The movement for open streets. Open Streets Project. https://openstreetsproject. org/

37 Adams T, Aldred R. Cycling injury risk in London: impacts of road characteristics and infrastructure. *Findings.* Published online December 14, 2020. doi:10.32866/001c.18226.

38 World Health Organization. *Community Engagement: A Health Promotion Guide for Universal Health Coverage in the Hands of the People.* World Health Organization; 2020. https://apps.who.int/iris/handle/10665/334379

39 O'Mara-Eves A, Brunton G, McDaid D, et al. Community engagement to reduce inequalities in health: a systematic review, meta-analysis and economic analysis. *Public Health Res.* 2013;1(4):1–526. doi:10.3310/phr01040.

40 Stokes, Gillian, Richardson, Michelle, Brunton, Ginny, Khatwa, Meena, Thomas, James. *Review 3: Community Engagement for Health via Coalitions, Collaborations and Partnerships (on-Line Social Media and Social Networks). A Systematic Review and Meta-Analysis.* UCL Institute of Education, University College London; 2015. https://www.nice.org.uk/guidance/NG44/documents/evidence-review-3

41 See note 38.

42 Cornwall A, Jewkes R. What is participatory research? *Soc Sci Med.* 1995;41(12):1667–1676. doi:10.1016/0277-9536(95)00127-S.

43 Oliver SR, Rees RW, Clarke-Jones L, et al. A multidimensional conceptual framework for analysing public involvement in health services research. *Health Expect.* 2008;11(1):72–84. doi:10.1111/j.1369-7625.2007.00476.x.

44 Piachaud, David, Bennett, Fran, Nazroo, James, Popay, Jennie. *Social Inclusion and Social Mobility.* Institute of Health Equity; 2009. https://www. instituteofhealthequity.org/resources-reports/social-inclusion-and-social-mobility-task-group-report

45 Kahn, Si. *Organizing, a Guide for Grassroots Leaders.* NASW Press; 1992.

46 Arnstein SR. A ladder of citizen participation. *J Am Inst Plann.* 1969;35(4): 216–224. doi:10.1080/01944366908977225.

47 White SC. Depoliticising development: the uses and abuses of participation. *Dev Pract.* 1996;6(1):142–155. doi:10.1080/0961452961000157564.

48 Katz R. Empowerment and synergy. *Prev Hum Serv.* 1984;3(2–3):201–226. doi:10.1300/J293v03n02_10.

49 Laverack G. *Public Health: Power, Empowerment and Professional Practice.* Palgrave; 2005.

50 Lerner M. *Surplus Powerlessness: The Psychodynamics of Everyday Life - and the Psychology of Individual and Social Transformation.* Institute for Labor & Mental Health; 1986.

51 Langford J, Clance PR. The imposter phenomenon: Recent research findings regarding dynamics, personality and family patterns and their implications for treatment. *Psychother Theory Res Pract Train.* 1993;30(3):495–501. doi:10.1037/0033-3204.30.3.495.

52 Labonte, Ronald. Health promotion and empowerment: reflections on professional practice. *Health Educ Q.* 1994;21(2):253–268. doi:10.1177/ 109019819402100209.

53 Berne E. *Games People Play: The Psychology of Human Relationships.* Grove Pr; 1996.

54 Kieffer CH. Citizen empowerment: a developmental perspective. *Prev Hum Serv.* 1984;3(2–3):9–36. doi:10.1300/J293v03n02_03.

# 8 COVID-19

The COVID-19 pandemic brought unprecedented change to the ways in which we live. The extensive scope and speed of change transformed the landscape of associational life. The need to reduce contacts altered our social norms in ways that have not yet settled. This offers the opportunity to reshape our relationships with each other, improving our health and our resilience for the challenges ahead. COVID-19 has been an important stress test showing the fragility of some systems.

Lockdown brought a stillness that many had not felt for some time, across communities, countries and worldwide. Breaks to routines brought people to new activities and ways of working. Global carbon dioxide emissions fell by 8 per cent in the first wave,[1] and an alternative, slower way of life emerged for many. Nature became more visible as the frantic pace of life faltered. Birdsong swiftly adapted to become more complex, enabling better communication over greater distances.[2] Human communication similarly had to adapt quickly. The rapid deployment of remote working allowed mobilisation and the safe continuation of services, and many workplaces have stayed virtual, reducing emissions, but working remotely does not generate the same social capital that thrives in workplaces and third places.

As the floodwaters of COVID-19 rise and subside, we are left with the detritus of our previous way of life. The pandemic stress-tested our systems, and showed up any deficiencies in resilience and adaptability. Those organisations able to respond most nimbly became stronger. A degree of pressure is important to enhance organisational resilience, bonds forged in fire being stronger. The increased capability that stressors bring is known as *antifragility*. Too much stress overwhelms, but not enough is similarly harmful, by failing to generate strengthening responses. Exactly the same happens with broken bones, which need stresses in order to remodel effectively.

COVID-19 became a significant turning point in the ways communities respond. The first lockdown showed beyond doubt the primacy of communities. This 're-wilding' of communities has allowed more responsive systems to thrive.[3] 'Social distancing' was an unfortunate phrase when physical distancing but social togetherness were needed.

The most urgent requirement was to support people who needed to isolate, ensuring access to food and medicines. This required agile, flexible working,

DOI: 10.4324/9781003391784-9

and communities stepped up to fill the need. Mutual support groups sprang up at local and hyperlocal scale. Community responses varied, according to the social capital already present. Neighbours checked on each other, ensuring that people who were shielding could get access to food and medicines. Social prescribers and link workers in surgeries coordinated with local VCS organisations to identify need and ensure help was available. Areas considered 'left behind' with less social infrastructure and higher deprivation had only a third of the mutual aid groups of other areas.[4]

---

**Box 8.1    Ross Good Neighbour Scheme**

Our Community Development Trust had been working on plans for a Good Neighbour Scheme, with neighbourhood buddies trained to provide locally based assistance. As the first cases of COVID-19 arrived in the UK, a frantic weekend saw the scheme rolled out early, offering food and medicine delivery to those having to shield. There were far more offers to help than people wanting befriending, but all wanted the same thing, to increase their human contact.

Locally it was hard to find roles for all the people who had volunteered to help, which was frustrating as there was a lot of goodwill and volunteers found helping beneficial. As well as mutual aid, volunteers welcomed people at the vaccination clinic, many of whom were leaving their houses for the first time in almost a year.

---

**Communication**

As the impact of this new virus became apparent, it was clear that urgent action was needed. This was a new disease with unpredictable behaviours, including early reasonable worst case scenario settings that were bleak. Lack of central leadership and preparedness made it clear there was no cavalry coming to rescue us; we were on our own. This was a new landscape, with real-time decisions needed and a lack of reliable information compounding the situation. There was little guidance, and waiting to be told what to do wasted time. Previous structures that required face-to-face meetings for decisions to be made were no longer fit for purpose.

In the first few weeks of the pandemic, establishing ways to communicate effectively was the priority. What information came through was either lacking or rapidly outdated, often with parallel but contradictory messages. It took some time for lines of communication to settle. Cascaded situation reports were the most helpful source of trustworthy advice, each service summarising the local position and any changes. Coordination between health and care providers, VCS, local authority and the new PCN structures meant responses were coordinated and more resilient, better placed to cope with surges and gaps in staffing.

Health messaging became critical, especially during the vacuum of information in the first few weeks. A dithering response meant official advice lagged weeks behind the dates when action was first needed. Local media were an important part of the communications strategy, able to give context and disseminate information in a trusted format. Clinical voices describing the reality of the pandemic brought home the importance of public health advice.

Meeting remotely has remained the default for many organisations, reducing both carbon emissions and the risk of transmission. While video conferencing offers a simulacrum of face-to-face meetings, the transactions are different. The side conversations before and after the meeting are often the most useful, clarifying or discussing ideas, but the ability to converse outside of the main meeting has been lost. The social glue of chatting about holidays and other non-work aspects is missing, making ties less robust. Starting remote meetings ten minutes early and staying online afterwards allows more of these extraneous but important conversations to occur.

---

**Box 8.2   Replacing the town hall**

Losing the ability to meet physically meant public interactions needed to move online. Churches and faith groups changed to meeting virtually, maintaining access for people seeking support. Without the social glue of contact, sources of information became more limited and vulnerable to misinformation.

The need to communicate advice and highlight help available led our Community Development Trust to set up a monthly live-streamed event, which continues as a platform for people active in the town to let people know what they and their organisations are doing, and how others can help.

A panel meets online for an hour monthly (using Zoom software, streamed live on Facebook), with viewers typing questions into the chat for the panel to answer live. Three or four guests talk for around ten minutes each, leaving time for questions in an hour-long session. Having one person to chair and another to field questions works well. The events are recorded so they can be watched back later.

Initially these live events were very health focused, covering COVID-19 and how to stay safe. Updates from trusted local voices helped to maintain community cohesiveness. Information delivered by local clinicians and public health experts seemed to cut through in ways that national media did not. The sessions were popular and provided a way to have 'town hall' discussions safely, with good reach into the community and the possibility for real-time interactivity. It quickly became a useful way for community groups to engage with people locally. Sessions were loosely themed to join presenters together, covering topics such as creative activities, wellbeing, social prescribing and pollution in the river Wye.

**The impacts of locking down**

Many pre-existing groups struggled to continue in the absence of face-to-face meetings. Even outdoor meetings were restricted, preventing safe access to exercise and friends. As conversations moved online, many of those in highest need of social contact were stuck on the wrong side of the digital divide. In 2018, 5 million UK adults (10 per cent) had not used the Internet in the preceding three months. Only one in two lowest-income homes have internet access, rising to almost all with incomes over the median.[5] Echoing the inverse care law, those in most need of connections are least likely to have digital access.

Physical activity decreased, particularly in young people, though not in high-income earners.[6] Those who remained active showed greater wellbeing and less anxiety and depression.[7] People showed more desire to interact with nature and gain the wellbeing benefits from being in a natural environment. Exposure to nature and greenspace during lockdown reduced anxiety and improved happiness and life satisfaction.[8] Even watching videos of natural forest scenes gave short term reductions in anxiety in people without access to nature.[9]

The first lockdown saw parkrun cancelled, not to return for sixteen months. This was national policy, as leaving decisions to go ahead down to individual parkruns could have encouraged travel to attend open events contributing to spread. Despite transmission being far lower outdoors, breathing heavily during exercise can produce a significant expired viral load, which could lead to transmission if in close contact. Closing parks and restricting exercise lost the benefits of being and meeting outdoors. For those with no gardens, the warm spring of 2020 was a particularly difficult time. Had the airborne nature of COVID-19 and the importance of ventilation been acknowledged at the time, some lockdown restrictions could have been avoided.

Loneliness was exacerbated by the restrictions, especially for those who were already isolated prior to the pandemic. By contrast, bonds that were already strong became stronger as households spent more time together. Older people showed a decline in mental wellbeing and an increase in loneliness. One million more adults in the UK were affected by chronic loneliness.[10] Meeting face-to-face protected against this, but virtual meetings actually increased the risk of feeling lonely.[11]

Lockdown was particularly hard for people living with dementia and cognitive impairment. The closure of meeting centres and bans on visiting care homes left many without opportunities for interactions. Any change to routine is disorientating, and being confined to rooms without family visits increased agitation and distress while reducing stamina and muscle strength. Masks and face coverings have been a crucial part of the COVID-19 containment strategy, but these reduce facial cues, which are crucial to those with hearing or cognitive difficulties, leaving more potential for miscommunication. Many people living with dementia showed worsening cognitive functions, while prescribing for behavioural symptoms increased.[12] Agitation increased the risk of wandering, which could spread infection. Rising anxiety, depression and apathy also caused stress to caregivers, compounded by a lack of external or respite care.

## Social capital and COVID-19

Social capital in the UK increased initially as a result of the pandemic, bonds strengthened through adversity. Communities supported each other with solidarity and kindness. Despite fears of increased suicide rates, countries saw reductions or no increase,[13] as Durkheim predicted over a century ago. As with other emergencies, solidarity behaviours tend to wane over time.[14] Social capital needs upkeep to retain its value, but lockdown and restrictions have affected our ability to maintain our bridging ties. Students and younger people with newer ties found moving friendships online more difficult. Restrictions on weddings, funerals and other ceremonies lost opportunities for togetherness when marking rites of passage and the reconnections these bring. Weaker ties dissipated, leaving smaller and more homogeneous networks.[15]

A rapid rise in participation accompanied the start of COVID-19, people finding creative ways to express concern for each other. The story of how we made our way through is an important shared narrative of the sentiments of joint purpose which kept communities alive during difficult times. The outpouring of trust and resilience have uncovered latent reserves of social capital. There have always been innumerable acts of kindness going on all around us, but COVID-19 has made these more visible.

Civic participation in the first year of Covid increased most in females, younger people and those of higher socioeconomic status, and decreased in people working in routine and manual occupations.[16] Neighbourliness improved, especially during warmer months with more opportunities for interactions.[17] Neighbourhood trust and feelings of belonging reduced, but trust in others generally increased.

The pandemic encouraged new people into volunteering, a rise in goodwill and increased opportunities lowering the barriers to engagement.[18] As older people and those with chronic health conditions shielded, volunteering increased particularly among younger people. One in ten adults newly volunteered, with more time to give due to furlough or redundancy. The desire to get involved during an unprecedented crisis saw an increase in social action (giving of skills or money, or participating in research) as well as formal volunteering through organisations. Participating gave a sense of purpose and of feeling appreciated, while providing routine and distraction from the situation. Volunteers enjoyed the experience, those with more involvement showing higher wellbeing scores.[19]

Volunteering was more common in key workers, people with mental health problems and those with higher educational achievement. Older people used volunteering to maintain social relationships when contacts with others were restricted. Social action was more likely in those with illness or disability, as people who were shielding still wanted to participate.[20]

The most affected economic sector was arts, entertainment and recreation, with nearly four out of five staff on furlough. The costs of venues are ongoing even when closed, making it hard for small organisations on tight margins to weather the storm financially. Expenditure on this sector opens up other economic areas as well as improving health and wellbeing, but the hole in council finances due to COVID-19 threatens future investment.

Access to education varied by income, with private school pupils twice as likely to have full days of teaching during the first lockdown as those at state schools.[21] A quarter of schoolchildren had no teaching at all, losing up to a twentieth of their entire time at school. Effects on families again depended on income, exacerbating the effects of inequality.

*Table 8.1* Impact of COVID-19

| | |
|---|---|
| Deaths | Two years after it reached the UK, COVID-19 had killed 161,000 people and infected more than 16 million. Each death lost an average of 11.6 life years for men and 9.4 for women.[a] 169,000 excess deaths were estimated in the UK by the end of 2021.[b] |
| Long Covid | The activities of daily life for 1.3 million people in the UK are adversely affected by symptoms of long Covid. 761,000 people have had symptoms for more than a year.[c] |
| Loneliness | The number of UK adults affected by chronic loneliness increased from 2.6 to 3.7 million, mostly affecting urban areas, those with more young people and areas of higher unemployment.[d] |
| Costs | COVID-19 is estimated to have cost the UK £394 bn in 2020/21.[e] |
| Council funding | There is a £7.4 bn shortfall in council finances due to COVID-19. The shortfall is putting spending on culture and leisure of £2.2 bn at risk.[f] |
| Education | Lost school time is estimated to lead to £40,000 lost lifetime earnings each, a cumulative cost of £350 bn across the UK.[g] |

Notes:
a  Hanlon P, Chadwick F, Shah A, et al. COVID-19 – exploring the implications of long-term condition type and extent of multimorbidity on years of life lost: a modelling study. *Wellcome Open Res.* 2021;5:75. doi:10.12688/wellcomeopenres.15849.3.
b  Wang H, Paulson KR, Pease SA, et al. Estimating excess mortality due to the COVID-19 pandemic: a systematic analysis of COVID-19-related mortality, 2020–21. *The Lancet.* 2022;399(10334):1513-1536. doi:10.1016/S0140-6736(21)02796-3.
c  Office for National Statistics. *Prevalence of Ongoing Symptoms Following Coronavirus (COVID-19) Infection in the UK.* ONS; 2022. https://www.ons.gov.uk/peoplepopulationand community/healthandsocialcare/conditionsanddiseases/bulletins/prevalenceofon goingsymptomsfollowingcoronaviruscovid19infectionintheuk/4august2022
d  Office for National Statistics. *Mapping Loneliness during the Coronavirus Pandemic.* ONS; 2021. https://www.ons.gov.uk/peoplepopulationandcommunity/wellbeing/articles/mapping lonelinessduringthecoronaviruspandemic/2021-04-07
e  Pope, Thomas, Tetlow, Gemma, Dalton, Grant. *The Cost of Coronavirus.* Institute for Government; 2021. https://www.instituteforgovernment.org.uk/explainers/cost-coronavirus
f  Local Government Association. *The Impact of COVID-19 on Culture, Leisure Tourism and Sport*; 2020. https://www.local.gov.uk/publications/impact-covid-19-culture-leisure-tourism-and-sport
g  Sibieta, Luke. *The Crisis in Lost Learning Calls for a Massive National Policy Response.* Institute for Fiscal Studies; 2021. https://ifs.org.uk/articles/crisis-lost-learning-calls-massive-national-policy-response

## COVID-19 and inequality

The unequal distribution of cases and deaths showed how strongly linked COVID-19 was to inequality and marginalisation. The link with ethnicity became apparent early on, with two-thirds of health and social care staff who died of minority ethnicity, three times the proportion within the NHS workforce.[22] Multiple factors led to this difference: higher exposure, worse health care, reduced access to protective equipment and the systemic effects of racism. Covid and the Black Lives Matter movement have underlined how racism is a public health crisis.

PPE (Personal Protective Equipment) masks are still based on the facial anthropometry of white male US Air Force pilots in the 1960s, which are less likely to fit women, Asian and Black people, increasing the risk of infection.[23] Pulse oximeters, which measure oxygen levels, are calibrated to lighter skin, which can hide a deterioration in the breathing of patients with darker skin,[24] racial discrimination ingrained even within clinical equipment.

Air pollution is also strongly associated with Covid mortality, even after accounting for socioeconomic status and risk factors such as smoking and obesity. Each extra $\mu g/m^3$ of small particulate air pollution increases Covid mortality by 8 per cent.[25] As London averages seven $\mu g/m^3$ above WHO guidance levels, this almost doubles the risk of dying for residents exposed to these excessive levels of air pollution. Toxic air compounds the risks from poverty and marginalisation.

COVID-19 case rates and deaths have been higher in more unequal societies.[26] The same pattern of increased mortality with inequality happened in previous epidemics such as Ebola, TB and cholera. Inequality rises after pandemics, but this is not inevitable; the Black Death killed so many that labour became scarce, giving the poor sudden bargaining power. Later epidemics such as cholera disproportionately affected the poor due to cramped and unhealthy living conditions.[27]

Occupation comprised much of the risk in the first wave of COVID-19. More than half of UK workers in social grades ABC1 were able to work from home during the first lockdown, compared with a fifth in C2DE.[28] Exposure to infection from service-sector jobs that were not able to be done remotely, together with increased crowding and financial stresses from uncertainty of work, all contributed to worse outcomes. Zero hours contracts encouraged employees to attend even when unwell, with delays of many months before widespread testing became available. Living in intergenerational households increased mortality, as did poverty and discrimination. The rapid provision of accommodation and testing for the homeless, preventing deaths and hospital admissions, showed how quickly this can be done if the political will is there.[29]

The initial dose of virus contributes to the severity of infection. High viral intake comes from being close to an infected person for a prolonged period of time. Activities which increase the expiration of virus such as coughing and singing are more risky than being quiet. In the first wave, the most affected were people in jobs working closely with others, especially those who were unwell, or in environments that were cold or poorly ventilated. Paramedics, health care assistants and nurses had high mortality rates. Outbreaks in meat processing plants showed how poor working conditions contributed to spread. Food processors, warehouse operatives and bus and taxi drivers were all at increased risk of dying.[30] Links to poor ventilation strongly suggested airborne spread was the main route of infection, but it took over a year for this to be acknowledged by authorities.

## Politics of COVID-19

At the start of the pandemic, the WHO declared that COVID-19 was not airborne, calling it 'misinformation' to state otherwise.[31] The Centers for Disease Control in the US took until May 2021 to accept airborne spread. Influenced by the cost implications of providing system-wide mitigations, this delay in acknowledging that COVID-19 is spread via air significantly slowed down attempts to mitigate spread using masks and improving ventilation. Encouraging hand washing and cleaning of surfaces pushes responsibility onto individuals, but providing clean air and ventilation needs systemic action and investment. While the SARS-CoV-2 virus that causes COVID-19 can be detected on surfaces, there is a lack of evidence that it is transmitted by this route.[32] It is far easier to blame cases on people not washing their hands than to accept the need for systemic modifications.

Shifting responsibility onto individuals in this way is a classic example of framing a problem in terms of individual behaviour. The way an issue is framed influences the solutions that are proposed. Shifting from an 's-frame' that identifies the need for systemic change to an 'i-frame' that emphasises the role of the individual helps to abrogate responsibility for effective public policy, moving to cheaper interventions which are politically less risky.[33]

The delay in implementing lockdown in the UK led to a far more severe first wave, although many lives were still saved by people locking down before it was mandated by the government. Locking down a week earlier would have prevented an estimated thirty-four thousand deaths and halved the time in lockdown.[34] Groupthink, aversion to risk and lack of preparation held back the government's response. The main concern of civil servants, few of whom had science backgrounds, was to avoid criticism at all costs,[35] a hallmark of a dysfunctional organisation. This was exactly what Dr Michael Ryan from the WHO Health Emergencies Programme had warned about at the start of the pandemic: 'Perfection is the enemy of the good…the greatest error is not to move, the greatest error is to be paralysed by the fear of failure'.[36]

Frustrated by the lack of contact tracing, some areas took matters into their own hands. Ceredigion County Council set up a local test and trace system early, which contributed to the lowest Covid mortality in mainland UK in the first wave of Covid.[37] In Sheffield, medical students took on contact tracing of inpatients with better engagement and results.[38] Councils were perceived to be far more competent than national government, and local approaches seen as more cohesive.[39]

Local newspapers were also a trusted source of information. Local papers improve community cohesion, civic engagement and participation, but have struggled to retain audience share against online media. In the twelve years before the pandemic, nearly seventy local newspapers across the UK had closed, with circulation down by two-thirds, a trend exacerbated by Covid.[40]

Trust in government reduces deaths,[41] but democracies had higher rates of both cases and deaths generally, as leaders needed to maintain support by preferring populist but less effective policies. Initial trust in the government approach declined significantly following some notable examples of leaders disobeying their own rules. Breaching of the rules by advisors, followed by the discovery that raucous parties had happened at Downing Street while the country was under restrictions, further damaged trust in the UK leadership.

Poor central decisions showed in the failures: squandered supplies, a flawed testing system and the spread of COVID-19 into care homes as hospitals were told to free up beds by discharging positive patients. The lessons from a 2016 pandemic simulation, Exercise Cygnus, had been ignored.[42] UK deaths in the first wave were more than twice the European average, due to austerity, inequality, poor pre-existing health, limited access to healthcare and a dysfunctional government.[43] Systems reliant on central control were left stranded, as shortages and staff illness took hold, a shock to those used to working in better resourced environments.

Slow access to testing and a poor contact tracing system hindered the UK response. Cronyism saw contracts awarded to close associates without experience, wasting many billions on expensive but useless PPE. The UK government's Eat Out to Help Out scheme in August 2020 spent £500 million subsidising the hospitality sector but is estimated to have increased new COVID-19 clusters by up to 17 per cent, which substantially accelerated the second wave of the pandemic.[44] The UK was fortunate to have competence in therapeutics development within the inner circle of government to guide vaccine procurement.

Populist governments, such as those led by Trump, Bolsonaro and Johnson, had higher COVID-19 death rates and excess mortality than equivalent countries.[45] Comparing the speeches of Prime Ministers Jacinta Ardern and Boris Johnson shows how the New Zealand premier predominantly used the word 'we' to position herself as part of the nation, while Johnson emphasised himself as leader, preferring the pronouns 'I' and 'you'. The UK approach was more authoritarian, commanding rather than creating mutual inclusivity, and shifting the locus of control from citizens towards government.[46]

Policy was inordinately influenced by a small coalition of academics who promoted the idea that allowing infection would bring herd immunity to allow the resumption of normal life.[47] This circular idea that getting infected is necessary to prevent infection does not make sense, especially when, as with other coronavirus infections, immunity is not long-lasting. Requiring those who are vulnerable to COVID-19 to isolate from society prioritises the needs of the well against those at higher risk. As happens with any successful public health intervention, the reduction in adverse outcomes from lockdown was ignored while the harms from lockdown were accentuated.

## Long Covid

This carefree approach to infection has left many suffering the long-term sequelae of COVID-19, sometimes following multiple infections. COVID-19 can be a very unpleasant disease for those who survive it. In the first year, one in five people still had symptoms more than five weeks after infection, and one in ten after twelve weeks.[48] Long Covid causes ongoing symptoms due to organ dysfunction, with limited treatment options. The loss of social identity from isolation and disconnection from others may compound the symptoms of long Covid.[49] Long Covid has been renamed post-Covid syndrome, professionalising and devaluing patients' experience of symptoms and claiming the territory for medicine.[50]

Although COVID-19 looks ostensibly like a respiratory infection, the microvasculature is damaged by thrombotic and inflammatory processes. Clots blocking small arteries prevent oxygenated blood reaching the capillaries, starving organs of oxygen and nutrients leading to impaired function. The SARS-CoV-2 virus enters cells via receptors found in multiple cell types including gut, lungs, heart, liver, kidneys, spleen, brain and blood vessels. Myocarditis (heart muscle inflammation), stroke, headache and lung damage are all linked to infection, fatigue, cognitive impairment and shortness of breath being common ongoing symptoms. Breathing difficulties are due to a mismatch between ventilation and perfusion in the lungs, preventing oxygen crossing over into red blood cells.

White cells have been found in brain tissue, bypassing the normal protection of the blood-brain barrier, changes also seen in degenerative conditions. The spike protein on the outside of the virus is associated with amyloid deposition, also seen in neurodegenerative conditions such as Alzheimer's disease, although the significance of this is still uncertain.[51] There are modest reductions in brain volume following COVID-19 infection,[52] with infection associated with a loss of seven IQ points on average, more than is normally lost over a decade.[53]

COVID-19 may well leave a longer-term cognitive burden, both from direct as well as social impacts. Reducing personal and community exposure by the use of mitigations such as ventilation and face coverings is crucial to reduce exposure levels and lessen the chance of infection and the longer-term sequelae of infection. Support for people with long Covid is inadequate, but online peer support remains a lifeline for many. The English National Opera has developed a 'Breathe' programme of exercises using singing to help people struggling with breathing following Covid infection, available online to people across England.[54] Activity and stronger local ties are likely to be helpful, so social prescribing has an important role to play.

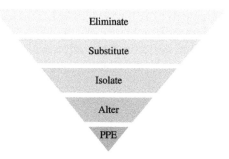

*Figure 8.1* Hierarchy of controls (National Safety Council, 1950s).

## Safely re-engaging with associational life

It is possible to regain our social lives while keeping the risk of illness low. Many people are still avoiding social activities due to concern about COVID-19. Social infrastructure that makes our shared spaces low risk by default will make our societies inclusive again to those at higher risk from infection.

Ventilation is the most important factor in reducing viral transmission. Outdoor spread is very unusual, as the virus mostly needs a confined space to build up to infective levels. Even small increases in ventilation give a worthwhile reduction in risk by diluting viral load. Opening windows stimulates air flow in a room, even if just for a few minutes every hour to reduce the potential buildup of viral particles.[55]

Where fresh air is hard to achieve, an alternative is to circulate room air through a filter to remove viral particles. High-efficiency particulate air (HEPA) filters have been shown to reduce viruses in air to undetectable levels.[56] Frequent air changes in rooms using controlled mechanical ventilation reduces viral transmission, with more air changes per hour further reducing risk. Changing all the air in a classroom twice an hour reduces transmission by 40 per cent, and by 80 per cent if changed six times per hour.[57] Corsi-Rosenthal boxes are cheap DIY approaches to circulating air through HEPA filters.[58]

Eliminating the hazard in this way is the preferred approach within the hierarchy of controls for managing risk (Figure 8.1). Sometimes this is not possible, so increasing levels of input are needed. Some hazardous products can be replaced with safer alternatives. If this too is not possible, the aim should be to keep people away from the hazard or change the way they work because of it. There will still be some roles which require physically dealing with the hazard, necessitating protective equipment.

Face coverings and ventilation remain the best way to prevent transmission by reducing inhaled viral load. For high-risk situations such as crowded public transport, good quality FFP (Filtering Face Piece) masks are effective ways to reduce risk of transmission. FFP3 masks have been shown to prevent viral transmission even in those working on high-risk Covid wards.[59] Masks are less effective for people spending hours together in the same room, where ventilation remains the priority.

Face coverings are inconvenient and impede communication, losing significant non-verbal cues and making lip-reading assistance impossible. Face coverings do provide a worthwhile reduction in risk, particularly when local transmission rates are high, but fixing the problem at source by reducing risk of exposure and improving access to fresh air makes it safer to meet again. Levels of risk healthy people may consider acceptable are exclusionary to those at higher risk of complications from infection. A change in our social norms will be needed to reduce the possibility of transmission, making our societies more inclusive.

Our infrastructure should be protecting us against airborne diseases. This means a systemic focus on ventilation in buildings to change air regularly. Quality filtering removes particulates as well as reducing viral load, though of course air should not need cleaning. Good airflow makes outdoor spaces naturally protected against airborne spread. The utility of these third places multiplies with seating, toilets and shade or cover. Siting spaces within natural environments also brings the benefits of greenspace. Developing these spaces is a key target for civic investment, given the significant return on investment. Future proofing where we live makes us more prepared for next time.

## Immunisation

Immunisation has been the mainstay of the pandemic response, although other mitigations are still needed. It is incredibly effective healthcare; more than ten thousand deaths had been averted within three months of starting the vaccination program in England.[60] Vaccination reduces the likelihood of hospital admission with COVID-19 by 80 per cent.[61]

Differing uptake of vaccines between groups has widened the inequality gap. The factors that predict vaccination acceptance fall along the usual lines of deprivation and marginalisation, but also political orientation. People with conservative political views are less likely to accept immunisation, especially when political ideology outweighs a broader sense of identity shared with others.[62] Hesitancy towards immunisation is more common with deprivation, in those with lower levels of trust in the medical establishment and in people of minority ethnicity. Adverse childhood experiences increase vaccine hesitancy.[63]

There has been powerful support for opponents of vaccination. Misinformation, spread particularly through social media, has introduced doubts about vaccination, instead opening up lucrative markets for unevidenced treatments. Motivations of the anti-vaccination movement are usually financial, political or based on the exclusion of others. These positions are amplified by misinformed citizens who are susceptible to manipulation of news, or who weigh the volume of debate as a measure of the strength of an argument. Media portrayals of situations typically feature two contrasting views, which acts to normalise and give excessive weight to fringe opinions, while the evidence is rarely considered. The opinions of the famous are valued over those with expertise, sceptical voices stoking a media fed by clicks. Social media amplifies fringe views,[64] cultivating doubt and persuading some that enough smoke must imply a fire.

The language used in communications affects immunisation uptake. The word 'jab', while conveniently quick, carries connotations of violence for some. Searches using the word 'immunisation' rather than 'vaccination' are less likely to lead to disinformation sites, making this the preferable term. Identifying with the local community is a strong predictor of immunisation uptake, mediated by a sense of duty.[65] The Latin root of immunisation, *munia*, means duty, representing our civic obligation to protect others, which is a strong motivation for people accepting immunisation. Appealing to a salient social identity rooted in community encourages prosocial norms such as helping behaviour and adherence to lockdown rules.

## COVID-19 and climate crisis

It remains hard to imagine under what circumstances COVID-19 will be 'over'. The important question is not when but how the pandemic will end. There will continue to be mutations wherever pockets of infection persist, so COVID-19 will not clear until the world has been immunised. In the meantime, reducing the risk and severity of transmission is both desirable and possible. Exacerbated by poverty and inequality, pandemics have rapid health, social and economic effects. The world has seen plenty of pandemics, but our damaging relationship with nature is amplifying the risk of future ones.[66] COVID-19 will not be the last.

There are parallels between the COVID-19 crisis and the climate crisis. The initial asymptomatic period made it hard to recognise what was to come, meaning that prevention and mitigation were not prioritised. Attempts to contain spread largely failed, making remedial action far more complex. Exponential growth is not intuitive to comprehend, and these crises risk runaway effects if not urgently addressed. We intuitively expect changes to be linear, but as tipping points are reached, outputs will change suddenly. An effective response requires widespread cultural and behavioural change by individuals and institutions, but long-term planning has been neglected due to the short-term nature of electoral cycles. The politicisation and polarisation of approaches has hampered our response.

COVID-19 showed how quickly governments can intervene, especially when this aligns with economic interests. Rough sleeping was almost ended in the UK during the first wave, but the political will to continue this dissipated quickly. Behaviours can change abruptly at times of disruption, but climate intervention needs to persist to be effective, unlike lockdowns, which were only ever temporary.

Wealthier countries have protected their own interests but will still suffer from the failure of a global response. Responses that are successful are held in little value after the event, as something not happening is far less noteworthy than the opposite. Interventions that work often generate significant backlash, as success becomes assumed while the costs are all too obvious. The wealthy insist on business as usual, and client media pass the message on without challenge. Funding for lobbying is hidden behind donor organisations, enabling donations without scrutiny. Simplistic and populist media messages are designed to downplay risk and undermine scientific advice.

Communicating risk clearly and consistently is crucial in balancing needs and responsibilities. Giving people the information they need to make decisions leads to better outcomes. The UK population were ready to lockdown sooner and for longer than their government believed they were able to. The spontaneous efflorescence of community spirit that arose through COVID-19 was not anticipated by those whose journey to power had been through competition rather than collaboration.

Governments have a tendency to restrict information during times of crisis. Controlling the flow of information feels a safer way to manage a situation. While this is ostensibly to reduce panic, lack of information is a more powerful driver of anxiety.[67] Withholding information will always reduce trust, and limited, delayed or contradictory official announcements sap confidence. The start of the pandemic brought a media diet of nothing but Covid, leaving very thin news bulletins and limited information spread across all channels. This information vacuum amplified all voices, so misinformation became more prevalent too.

## Lessons for the next crisis

The same patterns keep arising. Extreme weather events such as flooding are becoming more common and more severe. The best mitigation strategy for flooding is to increase the water holding capacity of land to slow water flow into rivers and reduce the peak of the flooding, protecting areas downstream. The same principle of 'flattening the curve' was the focus of the initial wave of COVID-19 lockdowns, limiting spread and allowing hospitals a better chance of coping with the unwell. As ever, it is better to improve our resilience and deal with the problem upstream. Working effectively and collaboratively is crucial for the changes that have to happen if we are to cope with the challenges to come.

COVID-19 showed the power of local action, which still prevails throughout our communities. Local responses are less visible than individual or political ones. Climate actions tend to focus on international negotiations, national policy and individual action, but this misses the efforts local communities can achieve, whether by improving cycle networks or running repair cafés. Climate action is often another outcome of developing community.[68] Above all, the learning and rapid development we saw during the first waves of COVID-19 showed the primacy of community. Building our resilience with subsidiarity and local networks fights both climate and societal breakdown.

## Notes

Links and additional resources for this chapter can be found at www.communityhealth.uk/8-covid-19

1  Tollefson J. How the coronavirus pandemic slashed carbon emissions – in five graphs. *Nature*. 2020;582(7811):158–159. doi:10.1038/d41586-020-01497-0.

2  Derryberry EP, Phillips JN, Derryberry GE, Blum MJ, Luther D. Singing in a silent spring: birds respond to a half-century soundscape reversion during the COVID-19 shutdown. *Science*. 2020;370(6516):575–579. doi:10.1126/science.abd5777.

3  Russell C. Supporting community participation in a pandemic. *Gac Sanit*. 2022;36(2):184–187. doi:10.1016/j.gaceta.2021.01.001.

4  Local Trust. *Communities at Risk: The Early Impact of COVID-19 on 'Left behind' Neighbourhoods*. All-Party Parliamentary Group for 'left behind' neighbourhoods; 2020. https://www.appg-leftbehindneighbourhoods.org.uk/wp-content/uploads/2020/07/Communities-at-risk-the-early-impact-of-COVID-19-on-left-behind-neighbourhoods.pdf

5  Office for National Statistics. *Exploring the UK's Digital Divide*. ONS; 2019. https://www.ons.gov.uk/peoplepopulationandcommunity/householdcharacteristics/homeinternetandsocialmediausage/articles/exploringtheuksdigitaldivide/2019-03-04

6  Mughal R, Thomson LJM, Daykin N, Chatterjee HJ. Rapid evidence review of community engagement and resources in the UK during the Covid-19 pandemic: how can community assets redress health inequities? *Int J Environ Res Public Health*. 2022;19(7):4086. doi:10.3390/ijerph19074086.

7  Wood CJ, Barton J, Smyth N. A cross-sectional study of physical activity behaviour and associations with wellbeing during the UK coronavirus lockdown. *J Health Psychol*. 2022;27(6):1432–1444. doi:10.1177/1359105321999710.

8  Labib SM, Browning MHEM, Rigolon A, Helbich M, James P. *Nature's Contributions in Coping with a Pandemic in the 21st Century: A Narrative Review of Evidence during COVID-19*. EcoEvoRxiv; 2021. doi:10.32942/osf.io/j2pa8.

9  Zabini F, Albanese L, Becheri FR, et al. Comparative study of the restorative effects of forest and urban videos during Covid-19 lockdown: intrinsic and benchmark values. *Int J Environ Res Public Health*. 2020;17(21):8011. doi:10.3390/ijerph17218011.

10  Office for National Statistics. *Mapping Loneliness during the Coronavirus Pandemic*. ONS; 2021. https://www.ons.gov.uk/peoplepopulationandcommunity/wellbeing/articles/mappinglonelinessduringthecoronaviruspandemic/2021-04-07

11  Hu Y, Qian Y. Covid-19, inter-household contact and mental well-being among older adults in the US and the UK. *Front Sociol*. 2021;6:714626. doi:10.3389/fsoc.2021.714626.

12  Suárez-González A, Rajagopalan J, Livingston G, Alladi S. The effect of Covid-19 isolation measures on the cognition and mental health of people living with dementia: a rapid systematic review of one year of evidence. *medRxiv*. Published online 2021. doi:10.1101/2021.03.17.21253805.

13  Pirkis J, John A, Shin S, et al. Suicide trends in the early months of the COVID-19 pandemic: an interrupted time-series analysis of preliminary data from 21 countries. *Lancet Psychiatry*. 2021;8(7):579–588. doi:10.1016/S2215-0366(21)00091-2.

14  Fernandes-Jesus M, Mao G, Ntontis E, et al. More than a Covid-19 response: sustaining mutual aid groups during and beyond the pandemic. *Front Psychol*. 2021;12:716202. doi:10.3389/fpsyg.2021.716202.

15  Long E, Patterson S, Maxwell K, et al. COVID-19 pandemic and its impact on social relationships and health. *J Epidemiol Community Health*. 2022;76(2):128–132. doi:10.1136/jech-2021-216690.

16  Office for National Statistics. *Social Capital in the UK: April 2020 to March 2021*. ONS; 2022. https://www.ons.gov.uk/peoplepopulationandcommunity/wellbeing/bulletins/socialcapitalintheuk/april2020tomarch2021

17 Abrams D, Lalot F, Broadwood J, Davies Hayon K. *Community, Connection and Cohesion during Covid-19: Beyond Us and Them Report.* Nuffield Foundation; 2021:61. https://www.belongnetwork.co.uk/wp-content/uploads/2021/02/Belong_InterimReport_FINAL-1.pdf

18 Jones, Dan, Jopling, Kate, Kharicha, Kalpa. *Loneliness beyond Covid-19: Learning the Lessons of the Pandemic for a Less Lonely Future.* Campaign to End Loneliness; 2021. https://www.campaigntoendloneliness.org/wp-content/uploads/Loneliness-beyond-Covid-19-July-2021.pdf

19 Boelman V. *Volunteering and Wellbeing in the Pandemic. Part 2: Rapid Evidence Review.* The Young Foundation; 2021:59. https://www.youngfoundation.org/our-work/publications/volunteering-and-wellbeing-during-the-coronavirus-pandemic/

20 Mak H, Fancourt D. Predictors of engaging in voluntary work during the COVID-19 pandemic: analyses of data from 31,890 adults in the UK. *Perspect Public Health.* Published online April 15, 2021. doi:10.1177/1757913921994146.

21 Elliot Major, Lee, Eyles, Andrew, Machin, Stephen. *Generation COVID: Emerging Work and Education Inequalities.* Centre for Economic Performance; 2020. https://cep.lse.ac.uk/pubs/download/cepcovid-19-011.pdf

22 Kursumovic E, Lennane S, Cook TM. Deaths in healthcare workers due to COVID-19: the need for robust data and analysis. *Anaesthesia.* 2020;75(8):989–992. doi:10.1111/anae.15116.

23 Chopra J, Abiakam N, Kim H, Metcalf C, Worsley P, Cheong Y. The influence of gender and ethnicity on facemasks and respiratory protective equipment fit: a systematic review and meta-analysis. *BMJ Glob Health.* 2021;6(11):e005537. doi:10.1136/bmjgh-2021-005537.

24 NHS Race and Health Observatory. *Pulse Oximetry and Racial Bias: Recommendations for National Healthcare, Regulatory and Research Bodies;* 2021. https://www.nhsrho.org/wp-content/uploads/2021/03/Pulse-oximetry-racial-bias-report.pdf

25 Pozzer A, Dominici F, Haines A, Witt C, Münzel T, Lelieveld J. Regional and global contributions of air pollution to risk of death from COVID-19. *Cardiovasc Res.* 2020;116(14):2247–2253. doi:10.1093/cvr/cvaa288.

26 Davies JB. Economic inequality and Covid-19 deaths and cases in the first wave: a cross-country analysis. *Can Public Policy.* 2021;47(4):537–553. doi:10.3138/cpp.2021-033.

27 Furceri D, Loungani P, Ostry JD, Pizzuto P. The rise in inequality after pandemics: can fiscal support play a mitigating role? *Ind Corp Change.* 2021;30(2):445–457. doi:10.1093/icc/dtab031.

28 The British Academy. *The COVID Decade: Understanding the Long-Term Societal Impacts of COVID-19.* The British Academy;2021. doi:10.5871/bac19stf/9780856726583.001.

29 More than 14,000 homeless people were accommodated in the first wave, which along with access to testing (UK COVID-PROTECT scheme) was estimated to have avoided 266 deaths and 1,164 hospital admissions. Lewer D, Braithwaite I, Bullock M, et al. COVID-19 among people experiencing homelessness in England: a modelling study. *Lancet Respir Med.* 2020;8(12):1181–1191. doi:10.1016/S2213-2600(20)30396-9.

30 Office for National Statistics. *Coronavirus (COVID-19) Related Deaths by Occupation, before and during Lockdown, England and Wales – Office for National Statistics.* ONS; 2020. Accessed June 9, 2022. https://www.ons.gov.uk/peoplepopulationandcommunity/healthandsocialcare/causesofdeath/bulletins/coronaviruscovid19relateddeathsbyoccupationbeforeandduringlockdownenglandandwales/deathsregisteredbetween9marchand30jun2020

31 Jimenez J, Marr L, Randall K, et al. Echoes through time: the historical origins of the droplet dogma and its role in the misidentification of airborne respiratory infection transmission. *SSRN Electron J.* Published online 2021. doi:10.2139/ssrn.3904176.

32  Onakpoya IJ, Heneghan CJ, Spencer EA, et al. SARS-CoV-2 and the role of fomite transmission: a systematic review. *F1000Research*. 2021;10:233. doi:10.12688/f1000research.51590.3.

33  Chater N, Loewenstein GF. The i-frame and the s-frame: how focusing on the individual-level solutions has led behavioral public policy astray. *SSRN Electron J*. Published online 2022. doi:10.2139/ssrn.4046264.

34  If the UK had locked down a week earlier, it would have prevented 74 per cent of cases and 34,000 deaths and reduced the time in lockdown from 69 to 35 days. Arnold KF, Gilthorpe MS, Alwan NA, et al. Estimating the effects of lockdown timing on COVID-19 cases and deaths in England: A counterfactual modelling study. Khudyakov YE, ed. *PLOS ONE*. 2022;17(4):e0263432. doi:10.1371/journal.pone.0263432.

35  Bingham, Kate. Lessons from the vaccine taskforce. Romanes Lecture; November 23, 2021; University of Oxford. https://www.conservativehome.com/parliament/2022/02/lessons-from-the-vaccine-taskforce-kate-binghams-romanes-lecture-full-text.html

36  Ryan, Michael. Daily press briefing. March 13, 2020; World Health Organisation. https://www.youtube.com/watch?v=AqRHH6e-y6I

37  Messenger, Steffan, Beltaji, Dana. Coronavirus: How did one county in Wales escape the worst of it? *BBC News*. https://www.bbc.com/news/uk-wales-53142088. Published June 24, 2020.

38  Foster R, Jones B, Carey I, et al. *The Successful Use of Volunteers to Enhance NHS Test and Trace Contact Tracing of In-Patients with Covid-19: A Pilot Study*. Infectious Diseases (except HIV/AIDS); 2021. doi:10.1101/2021.01.28.21250096.

39  Abrams, Dominic, Lalot, Fanny. *What Has Happened to Trust and Cohesion since Tier 4 Restrictions and the Third National Lockdown (December 2020 – March 2021)? Further Evidence from National Surveys*. Centre for the Study of Group Processes; 2021. https://www.thebritishacademy.ac.uk/publications/covid-decade-what-happened-trust-cohesion-tier-4-restrictions-third-national-lockdown/

40  Wilkinson L. *A Pressing Issue: Local Newspaper Performance and Local Election Turnout*. Plum Consulting; 2020. https://plumconsulting.co.uk/wpdm-package/plum-insight-oct-2020-local-newspaper-performance-and-local-election-turnout/

41  Zaki BL, Nicoli F, Wayenberg E, Verschuere B. In trust we trust: the impact of trust in government on excess mortality during the COVID-19 pandemic. *Public Policy Adm*. 2022; 37(2):226–252. doi:10.1177/09520767211058003.

42  Pollock K, Coles E. Mind the gap: from recommendation to practice in crisis management. Exploring the gap between the "lessons identified" during Exercise Cygnus and the UK government response to COVID-19. *J Emerg Manag*. 2021; 19(7):133–149. doi:10.5055/jem.0596.

43  Marmot, Michael, Allen, Jessica, Goldblatt, Peter, Herd, Eleanor, Morrison, Joana. *Build Back Fairer: The Covid-19 Marmot Review. The Pandemic, Socioeconomic and Health Inequalities in England*. Institute of Health Equity; 2020. https://www.instituteofhealthequity.org/resources-reports/build-back-fairer-the-covid-19-marmot-review

44  Fetzer T. Subsidising the spread of COVID-19: evidence from the UK's Eat-Out-to-Help-Out scheme. *Econ J*. 2022; 132(643):1200–1217. doi:10.1093/ej/ueab074.

45  Ritchie, Hannah, Mathieu, Edouard, Rodés-Guirao, Lucas, et al. Coronavirus pandemic (COVID-19) dataset. Published online August 25, 2022. Accessed August 25, 2022. https://ourworldindata.org/coronavirus

46  Vignoles VL, Jaser Z, Taylor F, Ntontis E. Harnessing shared identities to mobilize resilient responses to the Covid-19 pandemic. *Polit Psychol*. 2021; 42(5):817–826. doi:10.1111/pops.12726.

47  Zenone M, Snyder J, Marcon A, Caulfield T. Analyzing natural herd immunity media discourse in the United Kingdom and the United States. Sriram V, ed. *PLoS Glob Public Health*. 2022;2(1):e0000078. doi:10.1371/journal.pgph.0000078.

48 Office for National Statistics. The prevalence of long COVID symptoms and COVID-19 complications. Published December 16, 2020. https://www.ons.gov.uk/news/statementsandletters/theprevalenceoflongcovidsymptomsandcovid19complications

49 Van de Vyver J, Leite AC, Alwan NA. Navigating the social identity of long covid. *BMJ*. Published online November 26, 2021:n2933. doi:10.1136/bmj.n2933.

50 Canino, Lucas, Gainty, Caitjan. Long covid-19 sufferers were given a new name for the condition. Why it matters. *Washington Post*. https://www.washingtonpost.com/outlook/2021/03/22/long-covid-19-sufferers-were-given-new-name-condition-why-it-matters/. Published March 22, 2021.

51 Nyström S, Hammarström P. Amyloidogenesis of SARS-CoV-2 spike protein. *J Am Chem Soc*. 2022;144(20):8945–8950. doi:10.1021/jacs.2c03925.

52 Douaud G, Lee S, Alfaro-Almagro F, et al. SARS-CoV-2 is associated with changes in brain structure in UK Biobank. *Nature*. 2022;604(7907):697–707. doi:10.1038/s41586-022-04569-5.

53 Hampshire A, Trender W, Chamberlain SR, et al. Cognitive deficits in people who have recovered from COVID-19. *EClinicalMedicine*. 2021;39:101044. doi:10.1016/j.eclinm.2021.101044.

54 English National Opera. ENO Breathe Programme. https://www.eno.org/breathe/

55 Jimenez JL, Peng Z, Pagonis D. Systematic way to understand and classify the shared-room airborne transmission risk of indoor spaces. *Indoor Air*. 2022;32(5). doi:10.1111/ina.13025.

56 Conway Morris A, Sharrocks K, Bousfield R, et al. The removal of airborne severe acute respiratory syndrome coronavirus 2 (SARS-CoV-2) and other microbial bio-aerosols by air filtration on coronavirus disease 2019 (Covid-19) surge units. *Clin Infect Dis*. Published online October 30, 2021:ciab933. doi:10.1093/cid/ciab933.

57 Ricolfi, L. *Controlled Mechanical Ventilation (CMV) Works*. David Hume Foundation; 2022. https://www.fondazionehume.it/data-analysis/controlled-mechanical-ventilation-cmv-works/

58 Clean Air Crew. DIY box fan filters – Corsi-Rosenthal box. https://cleanaircrew.org/box-fan-filters/

59 FFP mask filters trap viral particles in an electrostatic mesh, reducing exposure by 95% (FFP2) to 99% (FFP3). Ferris M, Ferris R, Workman C, et al. Efficacy of FFP3 respirators for prevention of SARS-CoV-2 infection in healthcare workers. *eLife*. 2021;10:e71131. doi:10.7554/eLife.71131.

60 Andrews, Nick, Stowe, Julia, Ismael, Sharif, et al. *Impact of COVID-19 Vaccines on Mortality in England, December 2020 to March 2021*. Public Health England; 2021. https://assets.publishing.service.gov.uk/government/uploads/system/uploads/attachment_data/file/977249/PHE_COVID-19_vaccine_impact_on_mortality_March.pdf

61 Lopez Bernal J, Andrews N, Gower C, et al. Effectiveness of the Pfizer-BioNTech and Oxford-AstraZeneca vaccines on covid-19 related symptoms, hospital admissions, and mortality in older adults in England: test negative case-control study. *BMJ*. Published online May 13, 2021:n1088. doi:10.1136/bmj.n1088.

62 Fridman A, Gershon R, Gneezy A. COVID-19 and vaccine hesitancy: a longitudinal study. Capraro V, ed. *PLoS ONE*. 2021;16(4):e0250123. doi:10.1371/journal.pone.0250123.

63 Vaccine hesitancy increased fourfold in people with four or more ACEs. Bellis MA, Hughes K, Ford K, Madden HCE, Glendinning F, Wood S. Associations between adverse childhood experiences, attitudes towards COVID-19 restrictions and vaccine hesitancy: a cross-sectional study. *BMJ Open*. 2022;12(2):e053915. doi:10.1136/bmjopen-2021-053915.

64 Möller, Judith. Filter bubbles and digital echo chambers. In: Tumber, Howard, Waisbord, Silvio, eds. *The Routledge Companion to Media Disinformation and Populism*. Routledge; 2021.

65 Wakefield JRH, Khauser A. Doing it for us: community identification predicts willingness to receive a COVID-19 vaccination via perceived sense of duty to the community. *J Community Appl Soc Psychol.* 2021;31(5):603–614. doi:10.1002/casp.2542.

66 Bedford J, Farrar J, Ihekweazu C, Kang G, Koopmans M, Nkengasong J. A new twenty-first century science for effective epidemic response. *Nature.* 2019;575(7781):130–136. doi:10.1038/s41586-019-1717-y.

67 Drury J, Reicher S, Stott C. COVID-19 in context: Why do people die in emergencies? It's probably not because of collective psychology. *Br J Soc Psychol.* 2020;59(3):686–693. doi:10.1111/bjso.12393.

68 Webb, Jonathan, Stone, Lucy, Murphy, Luke, Hunter, Jack. *The Climate Commons: How Communities Can Thrive in a Climate Changing World.* Institute for Public Policy Research; 2021. https://www.ippr.org/research/publications/the-climate-commons

# 9    Planetary health

Just as our planet orbits in the 'Goldilocks' zone, neither too hot nor too cold but 'just right', our economy and resource use have to stay within certain boundaries. Too little economic activity leaves us unable to meet human needs such as education, housing, employment and health. Excessive activity pushes past the limit of what our planet can sustainably provide.

There are breaking points beyond which the sustainability of human life is threatened, occurring along nine 'planetary boundaries'.[1] Climate change, ocean acidification, depletion of the ozone layer, nitrogen and phosphorus fertiliser loading, freshwater use, land conversion and loss of biodiversity all have defined safe limits, which have already been exceeded for three: climate change, biodiversity loss and nitrogen. No safe limits have been established for the other two boundaries: chemical and atmospheric pollution. In these complex, interrelated, dynamic systems, pressure on one boundary influences the others. Keeping within these limits is necessary to maintain the unusually steady state of the earth's climate over the Holocene, the interglacial period of the last twelve millennia, when humans shifted from finding food to growing it.

The safe zone of economic activity, which stays within these planetary boundaries but allows sufficient and equitable resources to meet human needs, resembles a 'doughnut' (Kate Raworth).[2]

Human activity, in particular the unchecked release of greenhouse gases following the industrial revolution, is pushing the planet out of this comfortable and stable climate into the unknown of the Anthropocene era. Feedback loops such as the albedo effect, in which loss of sea ice reduces reflection of the sun's rays, exacerbating the warming effect, may contribute to runaway effects. Similarly, melting of the permafrost will release methane, which has thirty times the warming potential of carbon dioxide ($CO_2$). These 'tipping points' form discontinuities leading to abrupt changes and the risk of rapid breakdown as thresholds are crossed. Opportunities to alter course are quickly dwindling.

Healthcare is a major consumer of resources, and a significant contributor to emissions and actions that stress these boundaries further. Exceeding these

DOI: 10.4324/9781003391784-10

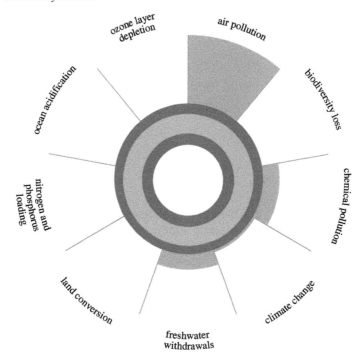

*Figure 9.1* Mortality impacts of exceeding planetary boundaries.

Worldwide, poor air quality causes 7 mn deaths annually; chemical pollution 1.8 mn; lack of access to safe water 1.6 mn; climate change 300,000; ozone depletion 49,000; and land conversion 8,300 deaths.

   Raworth, Kate. *Doughnut Economics: Seven Ways to Think like a 21st-Century Econo*mist. Random House; 2017.

boundaries leads to adverse health effects across populations, with the world's poorest most vulnerable. There are impacts on health across each of these nine planetary boundaries.

## Depletion of the ozone layer

The ozone layer in the stratosphere protects us from the sun, but has decreased as a result of human activity. Some sunlight is good for us, the action of ultraviolet light (UV) on the skin making vitamin D, which is needed for immunity and bone health. Vitamin D made from sun on skin lasts far longer in the body than that derived from oral supplements, without any risk of excessive dosing. Elderly skin needs proportionately more sunshine to make vitamin D, a good reason for older people to spend more time outside.

   The health risk to humans from ozone depletion comes from the action of unattenuated sunlight on our bodies. Reduced ozone levels have left us exposed to more ultraviolet light, which causes sunburn and other forms of cellular damage. UV light suppresses cell-mediated immunity, allowing cancers to develop and increasing the severity of viral infections such as herpes. DNA in skin cells is directly damaged by UV-B radiation, contributing to skin cancers such as melanoma, which are increasing as a result of ozone layer loss.[3]

Healthcare has been responsible for some of the damage to the ozone layer. Chlorofluorocarbon (CFC) propellants in inhalers were outlawed in 1989 by the Montreal Protocol. This change was unusually straightforward to implement, as it was supported by commercial interests; the main producer, fearing being undercut, wanted competitors to be forced to change as well.[4] Their replacement, hydrofluorocarbons (HFC) are instead potent greenhouse gases, with up to ten thousand times the warming potential of $CO_2$ and annual inhaler footprints of almost half a tonne of $CO_2e$ ($CO_2$ equivalent).[5] Newer propellants have a lower global warming potential, but the least environmentally damaging are dry powder inhalers. These are not suitable for everyone; propellant driven inhalers are easier for younger children and people with breathing difficulties. Switching just one in ten inhalers in England to low carbon alternatives would save fifty-eight thousand tonnes of $CO_2e$ annually.[6]

## Air quality

Pollution from particulate matter and exhaust gases is a major cause of respiratory illness. The coroner's report on the death of nine-year-old Ella Kissi-Debrah in 2013 was the first to list air pollution as a direct cause of death, with dangerous levels of nitrogen dioxide ($NO_2$) from the South Circular Road measured near her home in South London. Pollution levels are higher in ethnically diverse neighbourhoods and associated with deprivation,[7] multiplying other risks for poor health.[8] The Choked Up campaign raises awareness of the toxic impact on people of minority ethnicity.

Increased $NO_2$ levels cause respiratory illnesses, and are associated with poorer health and excess mortality, especially in areas of more deprivation.[9] Poor air quality in cities is hugely damaging to health. Ozone levels peak in cities around lunchtime, $NO_2$ levels during the evening commute. Peak ozone, particulates and $NO_2$ in London are consistently above levels shown to cause adverse health effects (Table 9.1).[10]

Particulate matter describes all non-gaseous content of air such as chemicals, droplets and solid particles such as soot. These are quantified by size, with fine $PM_{2.5}$ particles under 2.5 microns (micrometres) in diameter, and coarse $PM_{10}$ between 2.5 and 10 microns, roughly the size of a red blood cell. Particles smaller than 10 microns can lodge inside airways, while ultrafine particles ($PM_{0.1}$, < 0.1 micron) can pass across into the bloodstream. Approximately half the particulates in the UK come from human sources, such as wood burning and vehicle tyres and brakes, but road traffic is the largest contributor to poor air quality. Noise pollution from traffic meanwhile triggers chronic stress responses affecting cognition, mental health, sleep and cardiovascular risk.[11]

*Table 9.1* Air quality in London[a]

| Levels (all in µg/m³) | Background average | Peak | WHO air quality guideline[b] |
|---|---|---|---|
| PM$_{2.5}$ | 12 | 27 | 5 |
| PM$_{10}$ | 17 | 32 | 15 |
| Ozone | 40 | 78 | 60 |
| NO$_2$ | 28 | 52 | 10 |
| SO$_2$ | 2 | 3 | 40 |

Notes:

a  King's College London. *London Average Air Quality Levels*; 2018. https://data.london.gov.uk/dataset/london-average-air-quality-levels

b  World Health Organization; *WHO Global Air Quality Guidelines. Particulate Matter (PM2.5 and PM10), Ozone, Nitrogen Dioxide, Sulfur Dioxide and Carbon Monoxide*. Geneva; 2021. https://www.who.int/publications/i/item/9789240034228

Every 10 µg/m³ increase in PM$_{2.5}$ increases cancer mortality by 22 per cent and cardiovascular disease and stroke by 5 per cent.

Source: Wong CM, Tsang H, Lai HK, et al. Cancer mortality risks from long-term exposure to ambient fine particle. *Cancer Epidemiol Biomarkers Prev.* 2016;25(5):839–845. doi:10.1158/1055-9965.EPI-15-0626.

Yusuf S, Joseph P, Rangarajan S, et al. Modifiable risk factors, cardiovascular disease, and mortality in 155 722 individuals from 21 high-income, middle-income, and low-income countries (PURE): a prospective cohort study. The Lancet. 2020;395(10226):795–808. doi:10.1016/S0140-6736(19)32008-2

Human-caused outdoor air pollution causes around forty thousand deaths each year in the UK.[12] Particulates cause most of these deaths, along with other pollutants such as NO$_2$ and sulphur dioxide (SO$_2$). Air pollution reduces the average UK life expectancy by seven to eight months.[13] Fossil fuels are choking us.

## Fertiliser loading (nitrogen and phosphorus)

Fertiliser use has increased sevenfold over the last forty years.[14] Nitrates and phosphates are very widely used as agricultural fertilisers, but much is wasted, half the nitrogen applied to fields instead washing off into water courses, dumping nutrients into rivers, which damages aquatic life. Water companies externalise costs by using our rivers and seas as sewers, discharging 3 million hours' worth of untreated sewage in 2020 alone into our water supply.[15] The damage to ecosystems which depend on clean water is immense.

Nitrates block oxygen being carried in the blood, known as methaemoglobinaema. Maximum contamination levels of nitrate in water are set to protect against this, but while nitrates in mains water supplies rarely exceed limits, levels in groundwater are higher with nearly one in ten samples from boreholes and springs showing excess nitrate levels.[16] Formula milk made up with water high in levels of nitrates puts babies particularly at risk. There are health risks at lower levels, including neural tube defects such as spina bifida, and an increased rate of thyroid, ovarian and colorectal cancers.[17] Red meat increases nitrate risks, while vitamin C in vegetables seems to be protective.

The ecological harm from excessive fertiliser use also causes human health problems by boosting waterborne viruses and diseases such as cholera.[18] Blue-green algae (*Cyanobacteria sp.*) thrive in the presence of phosphate in water, especially when water temperatures rise, lowering oxygen levels, which harms fish and other aquatic organisms. The irritant cyanotoxins these bacteria produce can cause dermatitis and gastroenteritis. The harms from chronic exposure are not yet fully identified, but cyanotoxins can damage hormonal functions, liver cells and nerves.[19]

## Ocean acidification

Atmospheric carbon dioxide absorbed at the sea surface creates carbonic acid, making the oceans more acidic as $CO_2$ levels rise. Algae proliferate in these conditions, forming toxic blooms which worsen biodiversity and air quality. Ocean acidity accelerates the accumulation of pollutants such as mercury, lead and cadmium into the food chain.[20] The economic burden is also high; livelihoods in coastal communities rely on unpolluted seas. Fish constitutes an important part of the diet for more than half the world, but the quality of nutrition from stressed species is diminishing.

The oceans provide a crucial role, sinking a quarter of the world's carbon emissions, but are vulnerable to over-extraction. Ocean floor sediments are the largest store of carbon in the world, but are disturbed by trawling the ocean floor, contributing to acidification and releasing almost as much carbon into the atmosphere as global aviation.[21]

## Freshwater use

Over a billion people lack access to safe drinking water, leading to 1.6 million deaths globally each year.[22] One-sixth of the world's population rely on meltwater from mountain ranges, but declining water stored in glaciers and snow will see between 3 and 6 billion people living in water-stressed areas by 2050.[23] Climate change is making water supplies more vulnerable to flooding as well as drought. Water-related conflict has increased and will do so further as resources dwindle.[24]

Unless our trajectory changes, the areas affected by severe droughts will triple by 2040, affecting a third of global cropland and exposing 700 million people to droughts of more than six months.[25] Food insecurity leads to economic turmoil and deaths. Crop failures increase poverty and hunger, leading to social unrest, migration and conflict. Farmers adapt by shifting to less risky but lower yield crops, such as changing from maize to sweet potato, which is more resilient but has a lower return, reducing the food capacity of the land.[26]

## Biodiversity loss

Species loss presents a less visible risk to human health. Exposure to diverse macrobiota and microbiota helps the microbiome residing in our gut, lungs and skin to regulate our immune systems. Reduced exposure to organisms leaves the immune system less practised at recognising different molecular structures. Diversity at the macro-level reflects microbial diversity, which in turn protects against inflammatory disease. This is one mechanism for the health benefits of time spent in greenspace.[27] This 'biodiversity hypothesis'[28] recognises the interconnectedness of nature, explaining how our interactions with our environment work at a cellular level to maintain health.

A rich tapestry of wildlife around us seems to be good for us. Along with vegetation cover, abundance and diversity of visible bird species is associated with better mental health.[29] Many of the medicines used today are derived from nature, and although there are species producing biologically active compounds which have potential as treatments, habitat loss threatens their viability.[30] Wider biodiversity reduces the risk from 'reservoir hosts', species such as rodents who are resilient to human influence and form an ongoing source of animal to human (zoonotic) infection.[31] Action to protect biodiversity will be more expensive if delayed; a further decade of inaction will double the social cost (to US$15 tn).[32]

## Land conversion

Increasing appropriation of land by humans has health impacts due to effects on biodiversity, deforestation, water use and pollution. Fragmentation of land into smaller, divided plots makes predator territories less viable, imbalancing other species and lessening biodiversity. Field monocultures discourage pollinators while being more susceptible to pests. Many plants rely on cold weather to reduce pests and encourage vernalisation, flowering triggered by a cold spell. Climate change is putting our food security at risk.

The spread of human activity has reduced buffer zones around remote ecosystems, increasing exposure to animals carrying zoonotic pathogens. Viruses such as avian and swine flu can jump species, especially when people and animals are crowded together. The SARS-CoV-2 virus which causes COVID-19 is thought to have started in a live animal market. Encroachment of agricultural land by deforestation and road building have increased the risk of infections such as Lyme disease, Nipah virus and cryptosporidiosis.[33] Mining accumulates pollutants and increases breeding sites for disease vectors such as mosquitos.

Changes in land use inexorably push people towards urban centres. This can be to escape the effects of conflict or disasters, or in a search for opportunities and employment. Urbanisation has negative health effects, not just from traffic, pollution and crowding leading to increased disease transmission, but also from loneliness and isolation. Cities are hotter due to trapped air causing 'urban heat island' effects, and dark surfaces absorbing more heat, which together with a lack of vegetation raises temperatures up by 1–3°C and up to 12°C in extreme cases.[34] Parks and trees create a 'park cool island' effect which reduces temperatures by a few degrees, generating a gentle cooling night-time breeze in surrounding areas.

While trees are good for health, they can have variable effects on air quality, both of particulates and allergens. Trees and other vegetation help protect against the effect of pollution, with barriers such as hedges halving exposure to pollutants.[35] Of street trees native to the UK, hawthorn, field maple and alder have the highest air quality benefit.[36] Male trees have been preferred by planners to avoid the costs of clearing fruits and seeds, but the allergic burden of pollen to residents more than outweighs any cost savings.

## Chemical pollution

Many pollutants are known to be damaging to humans, with hundreds of toxic chemicals recognised. Toxins such as methylmercury in industrial waste caused widespread neurological manifestations for thousands of people in Japan (Minamata disease). It is possible for pollutants to cross the placenta, triggering genetic susceptibilities in one in four people with developmental disabilities.[37] Lead is a neurotoxin which can enter the brain, causing damage especially in the developing brains of children. Higher levels of lead are associated with lower intelligence and increased impulsivity, including violent crime. The homicide rate in the US later fell after lead was removed from vehicle fuel, more than halving violent crime.[38]

The healthcare system generates pollutants, predominantly from the production and disposal of medicines. Pollutants in wastewater are treated by adsorption onto activated sludge, though removal of these active pharmaceutical ingredients varies, with much medication still entering groundwater supplies in unmetabolised form. Medicines that are flushed away rather than disposed of properly at a pharmacy cause harm; our rivers and oceans begin at our sink plugs.

High-dose antibiotics in livestock and contaminated sludge applied to agricultural fields are other routes by which pollutants reach groundwater. Oestrogen, beta blockers, macrolide antibiotics and anti-inflammatory drugs are widespread in rivers at levels likely to have effects.[39] Antibiotics in natural environments can reach levels sufficient to cause microbial resistance.[40] Some drugs, such as the antiepileptic carbamazepine, persist and are found in drinking water, though not at levels considered to have an impact on humans. Doses in effluent can reach much higher levels, and antidepressants have been found in concentrated levels in fish, adversely affecting escape behaviour from predators.[41]

Reducing unnecessary prescribing is the best way to reduce the impact of our medicines on our environment, by being open to non-pharmacological treatments, reducing inappropriate usage and promoting the safe disposal of medicines.

## Climate change

Carbon dioxide levels are higher now than they have been at any time in the last 2 million years,[42] while other greenhouse gases such as methane and nitrous oxide have increased dramatically due to human activity. As a result, global surface temperatures in the last decade have increased by more than one degree, compared to the years between 1850 and 1900. The effects of the climate and ecological emergency are already here, climate change unequivocally proven to be due to human activity. Only urgent, sustained worldwide action will avoid a temperature rise that will cause massive impacts on health and the sustainability of life as we currently know it.

Since 1850, humans have emitted 2,390 gigatonnes of carbon dioxide ($GtCO_2$), a gigatonne being a billion tonnes. By 2020 we had a budget of 400 $GtCO_2$ left to have a reasonable chance of staying below 1.5°C of warming. As the world emitted 36 $GtCO_2$ in the year 2019,[43] our remaining carbon budget will have run out by the end of the decade. Temperatures will continue to rise quickly until we achieve net zero emissions. We are very rapidly losing the chance to change direction.

Lower-income countries have contributed least to the causes of climate change, but will be most affected by the consequences.[44] Poorer people are more exposed and less resilient to the effects of climate breakdown. Low-income African countries will lose five hundred times more life years than those in Europe as a result.[45] Inequalities as a result of climate change persist at more local levels; poorer people have fewer assets to build resilience, and are more likely to live in areas vulnerable to flooding.[46] Women are less mobile than men due to care commitments, making them more vulnerable to displacement and subsequent exploitation.

## Health effects of climate change

Climate change will affect health in a number of ways, some less directly than others, with immediate and delayed effects. The health impacts of air pollution are insidious and modulated by other health determinants. Extreme weather events will become increasingly common with global warming threatening food supplies, jobs, shelter and leading to population displacement. Hurricanes, landslides and wildfires risk life and health at the time and afterwards, from disrupted sanitation and infrastructure. Every half a degree rise in temperature significantly increases the risk of heat waves, flooding and drought. The frequency of extreme heat events will increase exponentially as temperatures rise.[47] Any reductions in winter mortality at higher latitudes are far outweighed by harmful effects, which disproportionately impact the poor.

Sea levels will continue to rise whatever mitigations are put in place, due to warming of the deeper oceans, but whether a two-metre rise in sea level takes two millennia or happens within the lifetime of our children is still within our control. Tidal surges lead to salinisation of fresh water supplies, losing agricultural land to the sea. Interruptions to food supplies bring malnutrition and susceptibility to other illnesses. Sea level rises will cause the displacement of large swathes of the population from coastal regions.

Rising temperatures may increase the range of vector-borne diseases such as dengue fever[48] and malaria, though the factors influencing transmission are complex and dynamic. This makes it hard to predict to what extent cases will increase, especially when human factors such as population movement and disease control are taken into account. More people will be at risk of malaria due to population increases and higher land in Africa becoming susceptible.[49] Climate change will force pathogens and people closer together and weaken resistance to disease from other stresses.[50] Pathogens such as anthrax, smallpox and the 1918 'Spanish' influenza virus may be uncovered as permafrost melts.[51]

Climate-related eco-anxiety is increasingly common especially among young people, who are rightly concerned about the state of the world they are inheriting. *Solastalgia* describes a sense of loss from the degradation of one's local environment. Mental health is worsened by climate change, with suicide rates increasing by 1 per cent with every degree rise above a temperature threshold.[52] People with mental health conditions are more vulnerable to heat-wave deaths. The psychological aspects of disasters affect far more people than the physical effects. Displaced people lose not just their homes but their cultural identities, connectedness and social support (see Table 9.2).

## Do no harm – the impact of healthcare

The sheer scale of healthcare puts it in a position to make a significant difference, making up 11 per cent of emissions, half a tonne of $CO_2$ per person each year in England (see Table 9.3).[53] Decarbonising the energy used has brought about the most significant reduction in emissions, which have fallen

*Table 9.2* Population impacts of climate change

| | |
|---|---|
| Deaths | More than 300,000 people already die each year from the impact of climate change, a death toll which will increase to 4.6 million by 2100.[a] |
| Temperatures | By 2030, temperatures will be above the threshold for working for 400 million people, with heat stresses above the threshold for survivability for 10 million.[b] |
| Infections | 2 billion more people could be exposed to dengue fever by 2080.[c] |
| Displacement | 26 million people had already been displaced by climate change by 2009, the majority due to slow encroachment such as desertification.[d] 230 million people live less than a metre above the current high tide level. |

Notes:
a Bressler RD. The mortality cost of carbon. *Nat Commun.* 2021;12(1):4467. doi:10.1038/s41467-021-24487-w.
b Quiggin, Daniel, De Meyer, Kris, Hubble-Rose, Lucy, Froggatt, Antony. *Climate Change Risk Assessment 2021.* Chatham House; 2021. https://www.chathamhouse.org/2021/09/climate-change-risk-assessment-2021
c Hales S, de Wet N, Maindonald J, Woodward A. Potential effect of population and climate changes on global distribution of dengue fever: an empirical model. *The Lancet.* 2002;360(9336):830–834. doi:10.1016/S0140-6736(02)09964-6.
d Desai, Nitin, Egeland, Jan, Huq, Saleemul, et al. *Human Impact Report: Climate Change — the Anatomy of a Silent Crisis.* Global Humanitarian Forum; 2009. https://www.ghf-ge.org/human-impact-report.pdf

*Table 9.3* Healthcare carbon footprints[a,b,c,d,e,f,g]

| | | |
|---|---|---|
| Blood test | 0.1 kg | predominantly from sample collection |
| General anaesthetic | 4.5 kg | per hour, using sevoflurane |
| Inhalers | < 2 kg | per inhaler, dry powder |
| | 9–20 kg | per inhaler, norflurane propellant |
| | 28–34 kg | per inhaler, apaflurane propellant |
| Analgesia | 0.2 kg | infusion of 100 mg morphine |
| Haemodialysis | 24.5 kg | for one 4-hour session |
| Outpatient appointment | 66–76 kg | 66 kg for primary care, 76 kg for an outpatient appointment |
| Inpatient stay | 125 kg | per bed day |
| Total of NHS, social care and public health | 540 kg | annually per person |
| Total NHS emissions (England) | 25 MtCO₂e | 62% from supply chain, 24% delivery of care, 10% from staff and patient travel |
| Global footprint of surgical activity | 4.4 MtCO₂ | anaesthetic gases can have 50,000 times the global warming potential of $CO_2$ |

Notes:

a Tennison I, Roschnik S, Ashby B, et al. Health care's response to climate change: a carbon footprint assessment of the NHS in England. *Lancet Planet Health*. 2021;5(2):e84–e92. doi:10.1016/S2542-5196(20)30271-0.

b McAlister S, Barratt AL, Bell KJ, McGain F. The carbon footprint of pathology testing. *Med J Aust*. 2020;212(8):377–382. doi:10.5694/mja2.50583.

c Sherman J, Le C, Lamers V, Eckelman M. Life cycle greenhouse gas emissions of anesthetic drugs. *Anesth Analg*. 2012;114(5):1086–1090. doi:10.1213/ANE.0b013e31824f6940.

d Smith, James, Bansal, Aarti, Barron-Snowdon, Joe, Keeley, Duncan, Wilkinson, Alex. *How to Reduce the Carbon Footprint of Inhaler Prescribing: A Guide for Healthcare Professionals in the UK*. Greener Practice; 2021. https://www.greenerpractice.co.uk/information-and-resources/clinical-considerations/guide-to-reducing-the-carbon-footprint-of-inhaler-prescribing/

e Connor A, Lillywhite R, Cooke MW. The carbon footprints of home and in-center maintenance hemodialysis in the United Kingdom. *Hemodial Int*. 2011;15(1):39–51. doi:10.1111/j.1542-4758.2010.00523.x.

f Andersen MPS, Sander SP, Nielsen OJ, Wagner DS, Sanford TJ, Wallington TJ. Inhalation anaesthetics and climate change. *Br J Anaesth*. 2010;105(6):760–766. doi:10.1093/bja/aeq259.

g McAlister S, Ou Y, Neff E, et al. The environmental footprint of morphine: a life cycle assessment from opium poppy farming to the packaged drug. *BMJ Open*. 2016;6(10):e013302. doi:10.1136/bmjopen-2016-013302.

by a third since 1990. Hospital emissions are mostly due to staff and patient travel and energy use in buildings. Medical procedures use a lot of materials, much of which are single use due to concerns about transmitting prion diseases such as Creutzfeldt-Jakob disease (CJD). Recycling equipment and consumables reduces emissions by only 5 per cent.[54]

Pharmaceuticals make up the highest proportion of emissions from clinical aspects of care. Life cycle assessments measure the impact of each stage of production. Making and processing medications contributes only a small part of emissions, as the majority of the impact comes from sterilisation and packing.[55] The climate effect of medications should be documented within formularies alongside side effects and other data.

Overprescribing, routine ordering and unnecessary dispensing contribute significantly to emissions. Non-pharmacological treatments reduce emissions but may be less acceptable to physician and patient. Once dispensed, medicines cannot be reused for another patient, which is hugely wasteful. Many medications retain potency for longer than their use-by dates,[56] and a more flexible approach is needed to reduce waste. New legislation in 2011 blocked charities such as Intercare collecting unopened returned medicines for reuse in lower-income countries.

The most effective way to reduce the footprint of medical procedures and operations is to avoid unnecessary medical care. Gallbladders and wombs, tonsils and appendices can often be safely left in place, but have all been removed in numbers far higher than the evidence justifies. Unnecessary or duplicated investigations are ordered for fear of litigation or due to the lack of shared records. Medical systems funded according to activity have little incentive to restrict interventions to those patients in whom the benefits clearly outweigh the possible harms.

Healthcare has significant purchasing power to select low-carbon options for transport and hospital food. The ethical imperative to reduce preventable mortality and morbidity means health workers have a duty to engage with upstream efforts to mitigate climate change. Health professionals are well placed to act as trusted communicators to advocate for climate action.

Focusing on the health impacts of climate change seems to engage people more than the environmental aspects. Positive framing is more effective, so discussing the need for action in terms of the health benefits of mitigation works better than discussing the health risks of inaction.[57] Catastrophic framing is often counterproductive by leading to disengagement.[58]

## Costs of mitigating climate change

The costs of inaction on climate are far higher than the cost of mitigation. The 2006 Stern review[59] estimated that it would cost 1 per cent of GDP to stabilise emissions at 550 ppm (parts per million) $CO_2$e by the middle of the century, but that not acting will lose between 5 and 20 per cent of GDP each year. The mutually reinforcing market failures that have led to climate change can be fixed.[60] Carbon pricing is the single most effective way to protect health from climate change, but this alone is too slow a process to achieve the necessary changes, as infrastructure networks such as transport and power take decades of planning. The value ecosystems bring will only be taken seriously when counted within balance sheets.

Attributing a cost to carbon provides a way to quantify the wider costs of emissions, in ways that expose the scale of current subsidies for fossil fuels. The social cost of carbon reflects the damage caused by one tonne of $CO_2$ over the next century. This was initially set at US$50 by the Obama administration, but was cut dramatically by Trump, who ignored impacts outside the US.[61] A more accurate estimate is between US$100 and US$258 per tonne.[62, 63] A related health metric is the mortality cost of carbon, which measures the increase in deaths per tonne of $CO_2$. At present there is one excess death per 4,434 $tCO_2$, equivalent to the lifetime emissions of nine people in the UK.[64]

Carbon footprint calculators help to demonstrate which of our activities have the most impact.[65, 66] Changing to active travel, reducing meat consumption and avoiding flying make the most difference to emissions. While reducing our individual footprints will cumulatively make a difference, carbon footprints frame responses as being individual rather than systemic.

The number of Earths we would need for current activity to be sustainable is a helpful way to visualise our overconsumption of resources. People in the United States consume more than five times their share of the Earth's resources. The ecological footprint of the UK is 2.6 times a sustainable amount, meaning that 2.6 Earths would be needed to maintain the UK's level of consumption if replicated globally. Another way to show this is 'overshoot day', which is the date each year when a country has used up its fair and sustainable share of resources.[67] Worldwide, overshoot day is July 28. The USA and Canada have used their share of resources by March 13, and the UK by May 19.

The health effects of climate and ecological breakdown are rapidly becoming a major threat to health globally. Low-income countries will bear the worst of the impact, but migration, food insecurity and conflict will affect everyone. Investing in action on climate is cost-effective in terms of health, even before considering the wider benefits. Just mitigating air pollution recoups more than double the investment in health costs saved alone.[68]

Addressing problems over longer terms with cross-organisational budgets is cost-effective with better health outcomes. While many of the issues are systemic, requiring policy changes to protect the planet that is our home, communities are also able to influence local action to protect diversity, reducing emissions by adopting alternative, low-carbon solutions.

## Notes

Links and additional resources for this chapter can be found at www.communityhealth. uk/9-planetary-health

1  Rockström J, Steffen W, Noone K, et al. Planetary boundaries: exploring the safe operating space for humanity. *Ecol Soc*. 2009;14(2). doi:10.5751/ES-03180-140232.
2  Raworth, Kate. *Doughnut Economics: Seven Ways to Think like a 21st-Century Economist*. Random House; 2017.
3  de Gruijl FR, Longstreth J, Norval M, et al. Health effects from stratospheric ozone depletion and interactions with climate change. *Photochem Photobiol Sci*. 2003;2(1):16. doi:10.1039/b211156j.
4  Smith B. Ethics of Du Pont's CFC strategy 1975–1995. *J Bus Ethics*. 1998;17:557–568. doi:10.1023/A:1005789810145.
5  Janson C, Henderson R, Löfdahl M, Hedberg M, Sharma R, Wilkinson AJK. Carbon footprint impact of the choice of inhalers for asthma and COPD. *Thorax*. 2020;75(1):82–84. doi:10.1136/thoraxjnl-2019-213744.
6  Wilkinson AJK, Braggins R, Steinbach I, Smith J. Costs of switching to low global warming potential inhalers. an economic and carbon footprint analysis of NHS prescription data in England. *BMJ Open*. 2019;9(10):e028763. doi:10.1136/bmjopen-2018-028763.

7 Fecht D, Fischer P, Fortunato L, et al. Associations between air pollution and socioeconomic characteristics, ethnicity and age profile of neighbourhoods in England and the Netherlands. *Environ Pollut*. 2015;198:201–210. doi:10.1016/j. envpol.2014.12.014.

8 Marmot M, Allen J, Boyce T, Goldblatt P, Morrison J. *Health Equity in England: The Marmot Report 10 Years On*. Institute of Health Equity; 2020:172. http:// www.instituteofhealthequity.org/resources-reports/marmot-review-10-years-on

9 Committee On the Medical Effects of Air Pollutants (COMEAP). *Statement on the Evidence for the Effects of Nitrogen Dioxide on Health*; 2015. https://assets. publishing.service.gov.uk/government/uploads/system/uploads/attachment_data/ file/411756/COMEAP_The_evidence_for_the_effects_of_nitrogen_dioxide.pdf

10 King's College London. *London Average Air Quality Levels*; 2018. https://data. london.gov.uk/dataset/london-average-air-quality-levels

11 Basner M, Babisch W, Davis A, et al. Auditory and non-auditory effects of noise on health. *The Lancet*. 2014;383(9925):1325–1332. doi:10.1016/S0140-6736(13) 61613-X.

12 Royal College of Physicians of London, ed. *Every Breath We Take: The Lifelong Impact of Air Pollution: Report of a Working Party*. Royal College of Physicians of London; 2016. https://www.rcplondon.ac.uk/projects/outputs/every-breath-we-take-lifelong-impact-air-pollution

13 NICE Programme Development Group. *Physical Activity: Walking and Cycling*. National Institute for Health and Care Excellence; 2012:120. www.nice.org.uk/ guidance/ph41

14 Foley JA. Global consequences of land use. *Science*. 2005;309(5734):570–574. doi:10.1126/science.1111772.

15 Slack, Amy, Tagholm, Hugo, Taylor, Daisy. *2021 Water Quality Report*. Surfers Against Sewage; 2021. https://www.sas.org.uk/water-quality/

16 Drinking Water Inspectorate. *Drinking Water 2020: Private Water Supplies in England*; 2021. https://www.dwi.gov.uk/what-we-do/annual-report/drinking-water-2020/#private-water-supplies

17 Ward M, Jones R, Brender J, et al. Drinking water nitrate and human health: an updated review. *Int J Environ Res Public Health*. 2018;15(7):1557. doi:10.3390/ ijerph15071557.

18 Smith VH, Schindler DW. Eutrophication science: where do we go from here? *Trends Ecol Evol*. 2009;24(4):201–207. doi:10.1016/j.tree.2008.11.009.

19 Otten TG, Paerl HW. Health effects of toxic cyanobacteria in US drinking and recreational waters: our current understanding and proposed direction. *Curr Environ Health Rep*. 2015;2(1):75–84. doi:10.1007/s40572-014-0041-9.

20 Falkenberg LJ, Bellerby RGJ, Connell SD, et al. Ocean acidification and human health. *Int J Environ Res Public Health*. 2020;17(12):4563. doi:10.3390/ ijerph17124563.

21 Sala E, Mayorga J, Bradley D, et al. Protecting the global ocean for biodiversity, food and climate. *Nature*. 2021;592(7854):397–402. doi:10.1038/s41586-021-03371-z.

22 *Global Health Risks: Mortality and Burden of Disease Attributable to Selected Major Risks*. World Health Organization; 2009. https://apps.who.int/iris/handle/ 10665/44203

23 World Health Organization. *Protecting Health from Climate Change : Connecting Science, Policy and People*. World Health Organization; 2009:32. https://apps. who.int/iris/handle/10665/44246

24 Levy BS, Sidel VW. Collective violence caused by climate change and how it threatens health and human rights. *Health Hum Rights*. 2014;16(1):32–40. doi:10.1146/annurev-publhealth-031816-044232.

25 Quiggin, Daniel, De Meyer, Kris, Hubble-Rose, Lucy, Froggatt, Antony. *Climate Change Risk Assessment 2021*. Chatham House; 2021. https://www.chathamhouse. org/2021/09/climate-change-risk-assessment-2021

26  Desai, Nitin, Egeland, Jan, Huq, Saleemul, et al. *Human Impact Report: Climate Change — the Anatomy of a Silent Crisis.* Global Humanitarian Forum; 2009. https://www.ghf-ge.org/human-impact-report.pdf

27  Rook GA. Regulation of the immune system by biodiversity from the natural environment: an ecosystem service essential to health. *Proc Natl Acad Sci.* 2013;110(46):18360–18367. doi:10.1073/pnas.1313731110.

28  Haahtela T, Holgate S, Pawankar R, et al. The biodiversity hypothesis and allergic disease: world allergy organization position statement. *World Allergy Organ J.* 2013;6:3. doi:10.1186/1939-4551-6-3.

29  Cox DTC, Shanahan DF, Hudson HL, et al. Doses of neighborhood nature: the benefits for mental health of living with nature. *BioScience.* Published online January 25, 2017. doi:10.1093/biosci/biw173.

30  Chivian E. Why doctors and their organisations must help tackle climate change. *BMJ.* 2014;348(apr02 3):g2407-g2407. doi:10.1136/bmj.g2407.

31  Ostfeld RS. Biodiversity loss and the ecology of infectious disease. *Lancet Planet Health.* 2017;1(1):e2–e3. doi:10.1016/S2542-5196(17)30010-4.

32  Vivid Economics, Natural History Museum. *The Urgency of Biodiversity Action*; 2020. https://www.vivideconomics.com/wp-content/uploads/2021/02/210211-The-Urgency-of-Biodiversity-Action.pdf

33  Patz JA, Daszak P, Tabor GM, et al. Unhealthy landscapes: policy recommendations on land use change and infectious disease emergence. *Environ Health Perspect.* 2004;112(10):1092–1098. doi:10.1289/ehp.6877.

34  Saaroni H, Amorim JH, Hiemstra JA, Pearlmutter D. Urban Green Infrastructure as a tool for urban heat mitigation: survey of research methodologies and findings across different climatic regions. *Urban Clim.* 2018;24:94–110. doi:10.1016/j.uclim.2018.02.001.

35  Mayor of London. *Using Green Infrastructure to Protect People from Air Pollution.* Greater London Authority; 2019. https://www.london.gov.uk/WHAT-WE-DO/environment/environment-publications/using-green-infrastructure-protect-people-air-pollution

36  Donovan RG, Stewart HE, Owen SM, MacKenzie AR, Hewitt CN. Development and application of an urban tree air quality score for photochemical pollution episodes using the Birmingham, United Kingdom area as a case study. *Environ Sci Technol.* 2005;39(17):6730–6738. doi:10.1021/es050581y.

37  Grandjean P, Landrigan PJ. Developmental neurotoxicity of industrial chemicals. *The Lancet.* 2006;368(9553):2167–2178. doi:10.1016/S0140-6736(06)69665-7.

38  VerBruggen, Robert. *Lead and Crime: A Review of the Evidence and the Path Forward.* Manhattan Institute; 2021. https://www.manhattan-institute.org/verbruggen-lead-and-crime-review-evidence

39  Comber S, Gardner M, Sörme P, Leverett D, Ellor B. Active pharmaceutical ingredients entering the aquatic environment from wastewater treatment works: a cause for concern? *Sci Total Environ.* 2018;613–614:538-547. doi:10.1016/j.scitotenv.2017.09.101.

40  Martínez JL. Antibiotics and antibiotic resistance genes in natural environments. *Science.* 2008;321(5887):365–367. doi:10.1126/science.1159483.

41  Daughton, Christian, Brooks, Bryan. Active pharmaceutical ingredients and aquatic organisms. In: *Environmental Contaminants in Biota: Interpreting Tissue Concentrations.* 2nd ed. Taylor and Francis; 2010.

42  IPCC. Summary for policymakers. In: *Climate Change 2021: The Physical Science Basis. Contribution of Working Group I to the Sixth Assessment Report of the Intergovernmental Panel on Climate Change.* Cambridge University Press; 2021. https://www.ipcc.ch/report/ar6/wg1/

43  Ritchie H, Roser M. $CO_2$ and greenhouse gas emissions. *Our World Data.* Published online May 11, 2020. https://ourworldindata.org/co2-emissions

44 Costello A, Abbas M, Allen A, et al. Managing the health effects of climate change. *The Lancet*. 2009;373(9676):1693–1733. doi:10.1016/S0140-6736(09)60935-1.

45 McMichael AJ, Friel S, Nyong A, Corvalan C. Global environmental change and health: impacts, inequalities, and the health sector. *BMJ*. 2008;336(7637):191–194. doi:10.1136/bmj.39392.473727.AD.

46 Jongman B, Winsemius HC, Aerts JCJH, et al. Declining vulnerability to river floods and the global benefits of adaptation. *Proc Natl Acad Sci*. 2015;112(18):E2271–E2280. doi:10.1073/pnas.1414439112.

47 See Note 42.

48 Morin CW, Comrie AC, Ernst K. Climate and dengue transmission: evidence and implications. *Environ Health Perspect*. 2013;121(11–12):1264–1272. doi:10.1289/ehp.1306556.

49 Tanser FC, Sharp B, Sueur D le. Potential effect of climate change on malaria transmission in Africa. *The Lancet*. 2003;362(9398):1792–1798. doi:10.1016/S0140-6736(03)14898-2.

50 Mora C, McKenzie T, Gaw IM, et al. Over half of known human pathogenic diseases can be aggravated by climate change. *Nat Clim Change*. Published online August 8, 2022. doi:10.1038/s41558-022-01426-1.

51 Christie, Alex. Blast from the past: pathogen release from thawing permafrost could lead to future pandemics. *Camb J Sci Policy*. 2021;2(2):1–8. doi:10.17863/CAM.74501.

52 Lawrance E, Thompson R, Fontana G, Jennings N. *The Impact of Climate Change on Mental Health and Emotional Wellbeing: Current Evidence and Implications for Policy and Practice*. Imperial College London; 2021. doi:10.25561/88568.

53 Tennison I, Roschnik S, Ashby B, et al. Health care's response to climate change: a carbon footprint assessment of the NHS in England. *Lancet Planet Health*. 2021;5(2):e84–e92. doi:10.1016/S2542-5196(20)30271-0.

54 Thiel CL, Woods NC, Bilec MM. Strategies to reduce greenhouse gas emissions from laparoscopic surgery. *Am J Public Health*. 2018;108(S2):S158-S164. doi:10.2105/AJPH.2018.304397.

55 McAlister S, Ou Y, Neff E, et al. The environmental footprint of morphine: a life cycle assessment from opium poppy farming to the packaged drug. *BMJ Open*. 2016;6(10):e013302. doi:10.1136/bmjopen-2016-013302.

56 Daughton CG. Cradle-to-cradle stewardship of drugs for minimizing their environmental disposition while promoting human health. Rationale for and avenues toward a green pharmacy. *Environ Health Perspect*. 2003;111(5):757–774. doi:10.1289/ehp.5947.

57 Maibach EW, Nisbet M, Baldwin P, Akerlof K, Diao G. Reframing climate change as a public health issue: an exploratory study of public reactions. *BMC Public Health*. 2010;10(1):299. doi:10.1186/1471-2458-10-299.

58 Myers TA, Nisbet MC, Maibach EW, Leiserowitz AA. A public health frame arouses hopeful emotions about climate change. *Clim Change*. 2012;113(3–4):1105–1112. doi:10.1007/s10584-012-0513-6.

59 Stern N. Summary of conclusions. In: *The Economics of Climate Change: The Stern Review*. 1st ed. Cambridge University Press; 2007. doi:10.1017/CBO9780511817434.

60 Stern, Nicholas. The criticality of the next 10 years – delivering the global agenda and building infrastructure for the 21st century. Presented at: The Stern review +10; October 28, 2015; London School of Economics and Political Science. https://www.lse.ac.uk/granthaminstitute/news/the-stern-review-10-new-opportunities-for-growth-and-development/

61 Wagner G, Anthoff D, Cropper M, et al. Eight priorities for calculating the social cost of carbon. *Nature*. 2021;590(7847):548–550. doi:10.1038/d41586-021-00441-0.

62  Stern N, Stiglitz JE. *The Social Cost of Carbon, Risk, Distribution, Market Failures: An Alternative Approach.* National Bureau of Economic Research; 2021. doi:10.3386/w28472.

63  Bressler RD. The mortality cost of carbon. *Nat Commun.* 2021;12(1):4467. doi:10.1038/s41467-021-24487-w.

64  Ibid.

65  WWF. Footprint Calculator. https://footprint.wwf.org.uk/

66  Global Footprint Network. How many planets does it take to sustain your lifestyle? http://www.footprintcalculator.org/

67  Earth Overshoot Day. https://www.overshootday.org/

68  Markandya A, Sampedro J, Smith SJ, et al. Health co-benefits from air pollution and mitigation costs of the Paris agreement: a modelling study. *Lancet Planet Health.* 2018;2(3):e126–e133. doi:10.1016/S2542-5196(18)30029-9.

# 10  Sustainable policy

Our world is in a state of transition. Climate justice, and the time it takes to achieve this will define the future of our planet. An economic system reliant on perpetual growth is unsustainable and damages the health of all of us, even those on top of the pile. COVID-19 has shone a light on poverty, inequality and marginalisation, which are all associated with worse health outcomes.

There are few signs of health and wellbeing considerations in recent policy decisions. An extractive economy has pushed prices up and wages down. Britain leaving the European Union has reduced the available care workforce, including a predicted shortfall of up to 400,000 social care workers.[1] The least connected areas were most likely to vote for Brexit,[2] although the loss of EU funds will affect poorest regions most. Since Britain left the EU, productivity has fallen by 4 per cent and economic activity by around 15 per cent.[3]

A decade of austerity policies and neoliberal collapse in the UK has left the safety net of welfare nearer to the ground than ever, with those in work increasingly likely to be in poverty. Rising household bills will increase the cost of living and reduce disposable income. Vulnerable employment and welfare sanctions cause direct harm to health. Economic downturns have impacts across the health of the entire population.

## 'We've had enough of experts'

This quote[4] is so far the high water mark of political disdain for facts and objectivity. Politicians are certainly keen to avoid professional challenge. Following the evidence leaves healthcare entering the disputed territory between health and politics. Improving health means addressing the wider determinants of health, but the ability to influence these sits firmly within the political sphere. As Virchow said, politics is merely medicine on a larger scale.

The COVID-19 pandemic has shown clearly the tension between political decisions and the public health evidence base. Those who have advocated mitigations have faced opprobrium from the media and their politicians, who have consistently downplayed the health consequences of the pandemic. There are similarities with the way the gun lobby in the US has tried to delegitimise the voice of healthcare staff, suggesting clinicians should 'stay in their lane'.

DOI: 10.4324/9781003391784-11

Speaking out is a duty for professionals, when keeping quiet would allow institutional harm to come to those we serve. Recognising the corporate and financial interests behind current medical practice protects patients from overtreatment.[5] Developing critical thinking exposes 'institutional pathologies'.[6] Moral discomfort when values differ precipitates activism to transform the system.[7] Health staff are well placed to advocate for change, as health messages cut through; a public health framing for climate action elicits more support.[8]

There is a wilful neglect of the evidence base in current politics. Dogma trumps effectiveness, creating normative rather than representative politics. Just as effective healthcare ensures that treatment is optimised according to the evidence, policy could and should be based on effective practice. It is clear that better equality improves our health while policy optimised to the excesses of a few hurts the many.

Policy has become reactive, with a lack of a coherent central vision coordinating policy compounded by frequent changes in leadership. More extreme versions of policy are leaked, providing an anchoring point allowing for subsequent moderations to look like concessions, shifting the Overton window of possible policy to normalise these positions. Without joined-up approaches between departments at national and supra-national level, policy will continue to fail.

It may be politicians the country has had enough of. Devolving the NHS from political control would stop ideologically driven micromanagement distracting from more effective care. The same principles apply across multiple institutions, freed from diktat to respond better to the needs of the people they serve. But when did politics take on decisions about care?

## Welfare policy

Before the introduction of the welfare state, support was civic in nature, funded by philanthropy. Population growth and agricultural changes left fewer people needed to work the land, leading to increasing unemployment. The Old Poor Law required parishes to support people who were unable to work, after the dissolution of the monasteries weakened religious charitable support which had subsidised labourers outside of harvest. The New Poor Law of 1834 was supposed to unify the system and reduce costs. Tax to support the poor was levied by size of property, although the gentry resisted any redistribution of wealth.[9] About one in ten of the population needed help in any one year, though conditions in workhouses were often intended to dissuade people from seeking help. Friendly societies offered members a way to pool risk, but this function was taken over by the state as the twentieth century progressed.

Various legislation to protect workers was introduced, including the National Insurance Act of 1911, but the modern welfare state in Britain began in the 1940s with a series of reports looking at living conditions (William Beveridge). The Beveridge reforms addressed the five 'giants' he found: Want, Disease, Ignorance, Squalor and Idleness. These were to be solved by the government taking responsibility for addressing poverty, improving health and providing education, housing and employment, the cost to be shared between individual, employer and state.

Beveridge recognised that communities were better placed to identify needs and provide solutions. His report on Voluntary Action recommended the continued involvement of mutual societies, although this was overruled by the post-war government. Beveridge understood the importance of mutual aid: 'Voluntary action outside of one's home, individually and in association with other citizens, for bettering one's own life and that of one's fellows, are the distinguishing marks of a free society'.[10] Implementing the Beveridge report saw the provision of welfare shift from charity to state, but the model remained top-down. Paternalism lived on through policy: 'the gentleman in Whitehall really does know better what is good for people than the people know themselves' (Douglas Jay MP).[11]

Policy is susceptible to *lifestyle drift*, over time slipping from addressing systemic issues to highlighting individual responsibilities. At the same time, there has been a deliberate shift from citizen to consumer in the way we identify with public services.[12] Changing to a consumer model brought market forces into healthcare, in the belief that competition would improve quality and reduce costs. This commodification of healthcare has led to less continuity and more market-driven medicine, valued by activity, but increasing choice has not made services more responsive or competitive.[13] Choice predominantly benefits people with more assets, as it is social factors such as income and transport that influence the ability to benefit from choice.[14]

Community offers an alternative paradigm for care which moves beyond state and market.[15] Healthcare staff help this process by focusing on strengths rather than deficits, sharing data, and by being prepared to give up control. Primary care networks offer a way to involve citizens, working in alliance to create health.

## Is there such a thing as society?

The idea of society itself, the complex ties of relationships that hold us together, has been appropriated by politicians keen to influence the way in which we relate to each other. When the then UK Prime Minister Margaret Thatcher told a magazine in 1987 that 'there is no such thing as society', Downing Street was later forced to clarify her views,[16] explaining that to her, society was just a concept abstracting the need for decisions and action. Leaving things to 'society' was to avoid taking responsibility. Her next line is less well known, about how the quality of our 'living tapestry of men and women and people' depends on how much responsibility we each take. Her successor, Tony Blair, extolled the values of community, saying that 'our fulfilment as individuals lies in a decent society of others'.[17]

Blair's neighbourhood renewal focused on housing, environment and community safety, as the importance of social capital started to be reflected in policy. Regeneration was prioritised, aimed more at increasing economic efficiency than attempting fairer distribution.[18] Investment in supply-side measures such as education, skills and infrastructure was intended to lead to growth. Greater NHS investment reduced the mortality gap from causes amenable to healthcare, particularly in deprived areas.[19]

The Cameron government's 'Big Society' was intended to capitalise on the potential value of community, but the impact of austerity politics created the suspicion that this was a cover-up for communities being abandoned. 'The idea took hold that the government wanted communities to fill the gaps left by the retreating state, while the fundamental economic order remained in place, palliated by the efforts of volunteers picking up the pieces from a broken model'.[20] Instead, the country would be 'levelled up', in an attempt to repair the damage a decade of austerity policies had wrought.

Despite using much of the language of community development, plans for levelling up have relied heavily on external specialism, the antithesis of an asset-based approach. Grand offers of help are envisaged, generating social covenants with companies eager to provide the 'wiring of our social infrastructure'.[21] Volunteers are repeatedly described as 'harnessed', betraying a mindset that sees volunteers as a resource to be exploited rather than nurtured.[22] The colonial view of the gentleman in Whitehall persists.

Much policy is recycled. Closed SureStart centres are reincarnated as family hubs, and libraries reimagined as twenty-first-century hubs, despite the closure of a quarter of libraries and a £200 mn reduction in library funding over the last decade.[23] Competing and contradictory policies make for very ineffectual provision.

Central funding for local authorities fell by £18 bn from 2010 to 2015. A Towns Fund of £1 bn was introduced to compensate, but fell subject to political interference, as the vast majority of the money was allocated to constituencies supporting the government rather than addressing areas of greatest need.[24] Neither the towns nor levelling up funds are subject to local decision-making.

Investing in deprived areas reduces mortality,[25] but redistribution to address inequality happens least when it is most needed (Robin Hood paradox).[26] Higher differences in wealth bring status anxiety, driving a desire to acquire more. Inequality breeds inequality. Having more to lose makes people hold on tighter.[27]

The levelling up white paper's reliance on trickle down theories was described by Michael Marmot as 'inappropriate by an order of magnitude'.[28] The theory of trickle down is that inequality of income is justified on the basis that money eventually reaches even those at the bottom of the income gradient. In practice, surplus money attracts to other money and becomes lost to extractive wealth. The state's function is to hold the risk.[29]

Large reductions in taxes for the rich over the last fifty years have worsened income inequality, with little evidence of wealth trickling down. These do not bring economic benefit; tax cuts for the rich do not increase growth, employment or investment.[30]

The political leaning of government affects health outcomes. Democratic countries have longer life expectancy and lower child and infant mortality, while strongly right-wing regimes do significantly worse on all of these metrics.[31] Inequality is markedly reduced and life expectancy improves under left-wing governments, the difference being most pronounced in lower-income countries, partly due to higher numbers of healthcare staff and better nutrition. Conservative governments have higher rates of suicide,[32] a disease of despair. Deaths by suicide in the Soviet Union reduced during *perestroika*, the opening up between 1984 and 1990, but have since increased to be among the highest.

A punitive benefits system in the UK has led to repossessions and long waits for payments, forcing poverty and deprivation on the already marginalised. The rollout of Universal Credit is estimated to have led to sixty thousand extra burglaries and vehicle crimes.[33] Regressive cuts from austerity have impacted women most, contributing to worsening death rates in deprived populations.[34]

## Polarisation and anomie

Politics has become ever more polarised, driven largely by oligarch-owned media. Think tanks and lobbyists are influential without disclosing their funding. An industry built on harvesting clicks favours easily digested, attention grabbing stories, the junk food of media, with little fibre within the opinions on offer. Space or time to absorb the complexity of an issue is scarce. Neoliberalism is enshrined within every editorial decision governing the vast majority of news outlets.

Oppositional systems of politics have imposed a binary, dichotomous structure onto issues that are far more complex. The whipping system to ensure a party votes as a block undermines the responsibility of representatives towards the electorate.[35] This feeds a simplified and polarised narrative to voters, whose only role is to outsource decisions every few years. Participation is discouraged even at local levels of government, with citizen engagement sparse and tightly controlled. Standing orders and formal structures curtail the ability of citizens to speak at official meetings. This insistence on formality reinforces the power of those already in charge, who know the rules.[36]

Political polarisation as reflected in media portrayals is a thin veneer, as we have far more things in common than divide us. Political hierarchies are imbalanced; while politicians on the left tend to align with the views of their voters, economic values become increasingly extreme and less representative of voters as right-wing politicians rise within the party (May's law).[37]

Governance is increasingly foregone in the UK. Appointments on patronage have become normalised. Integrity is one of the seven Nolan principles for conduct in Public Office, ensuring probity by forbidding family or friends to benefit financially from decisions, but marking one's own homework circumvents this. The processes for PPE procurement were unlawful and

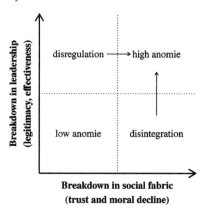

*Figure 10.1* Conceptual framework of anomie.

Teymoori A, Bastian B, Jetten J. Towards a psychological analysis of anomie. *Polit Psychol.* 2017;38(6):1009–1023. doi:10.1111/pops.12377.

strongly favoured people with close pre-existing ties to decision-makers.[38] Billions were spent on unsuitable equipment, using public finances to reward party donors and cronies. *State capture* describes the process of lobbyists and private interests influencing policy to gain financially.

Social disintegration, *anomie*, comes from dysfunctional leadership and the breakdown of social norms. Durkheim warned this would occur when industry became the 'supreme end of individuals and societies alike'.[39] An erosion of trust damages our shared ideas of ethical and moral standards. Disregulation, due to illegitimate or ineffective leadership, together with disintegration, a breakdown in social norms, leads to a shared perception of societal collapse (Figure 10.1).[40] The perception of breakdown alone is enough to trigger anomie, which interferes with basic human needs: meaning, self-esteem, connection and sense of control. As our social selves contract, we withdraw from the wider community to seek safer connections, damaging our interactions and our health.

## Meta-crisis

A lack of action despite the urgent necessity makes the climate emergency a meta-crisis of multiple, interconnected factors. Our inability to act in the face of threats compounds the problem, as we freeze in the headlights of the upcoming crash. Breaking our addiction to fossil fuels needs planning far beyond political cycles of a few years. The distance in both time and geography makes climate breakdown hard to envision; humans find it hard to visualise more than fifteen to twenty years into the future.[41]

A large amount of money is spent maintaining the status quo, though this spending is often opaque. Donor foundations hide the identities of those funding climate change counter-movements, bearing remarkable similarity to the funding streams of the larger conservative movement.[42] It is more profitable in the short term for the fossil fuel industry to fund climate denial than it would be to shift away from a carbon-based economy, despite their very prescient predictions about the scale of damage caused.[43] As with the tactics of the tobacco industry, the main aim is to introduce enough confusion and misinformation into the debate to disengage sufficient people. Scientific debate about extent is misrepresented as uncertainty about climate change, which seeks to create enough doubt to avoid taking action. This plays into concerns about government control or assaults on liberty, and helps embed climate scepticism within a wider political fringe. Bad actors can generate enough confusion to keep many from changing position.

The power of media to influence us is attested to by the huge resources behind automated social media accounts trying to disrupt, bully or curate a particular view. Social media can be a powerful empty vessel, full of sound and fury. Exposure to other views is outweighed by the desire for opinion reinforcement, which reinforces the 'echo chamber' effect.[44] Social networks give the impression of engagement, but online discourse is unidimensional compared with sharing the same space physically. The bridging potential of social networking sites can be very powerful with a wide reach, but translating ideas from online to offline is where the real wellbeing benefits start.

The rise of 'post-truth' forces questions about our relationships with empirical facts. The idea that all knowledge is socially constructed, with no basis in objective, shared reality, undermines the foundations of science. Conspiracy theories allow us to manage stress by offering a simple explanation for threatening events, which restores our sense of control.[45] Appeals to emotion overtake objective evidence, which is rejected on the basis of the cultural associations wrapped around it. This allows a murkiness around truth that hides attempts to warp and manipulate.

Recent politics has increased attempts at othering, reinforcing sense of identity by differentiating those outside the group. Inciting inter-group hostility breeds entitlement, hostility and resentment. Seeking privilege rather than equality, a belief that the in-group is exceptional but under-recognised constitutes *collective narcissism*.[46]

## Neoliberalism

The word *economics* comes from *oikonomia*, managing a household prudently. The concept originally referred to being sufficient, avoiding profligacy and engaging with public life.[47] Modern financial practice leans far more towards *chrematistics*, the gaining of wealth typically by maximising short-term profits. Neoliberalism has become the pervasive economic system, putting competition at the heart of our interactions, success measured by production and growth. Having enough is no longer enough.

Current fiscal policy strongly reinforces the gravitational pull of money, whereby the rich get richer (Matthew effect). The resources we are born to vary hugely.[48] This 'primitive accumulation' imbalances the distribution of money leading to persistent inequality. Capitalism explains this initial differential in wealth as being due to parsimony,[49] failing to acknowledge the wealth accumulated by colonialism, plunder and the enclosure of lands.[50]

Money that enters the corporate sector struggles to find its way back into a local economy. This wealth is extracted and becomes unavailable. New money created by quantitative easing is used to restore the balance sheets of banks, even though introducing money at lower income bands stimulates the economy more successfully. Trickle up generates more economic activity, as money circulates more times, but increasing the income of the poorest would undermine the demonisation of the poor as feckless, which is used to justify inequality.

Tax fraud prosecutions are declining; despite welfare fraud costing the Exchequer nine times less than tax fraud, there are twenty-three times as many prosecutions for welfare fraud.[51] Welfare fraud is often referred for prosecution, tax fraud rarely so. Encouraging welfare claimants to collect benefits stimulates local economies far more than reducing taxes.

Corporations acting purely in the service of shareholder profit has led to devastating waste. Externalising costs makes balance sheets look better and deflects the problem for someone else to fix, allowing more efficient wealth extraction. A company which pollutes rather than paying to deal with waste simply offloads the cost onto wider society. Shifting production to lower-income countries has similarly been used to divert blame for emissions onto those countries.

Deregulation offers a further way to decouple polluters from paying the cost. Water companies can continue giving out dividends without pressure to improve their infrastructure. Our society subsidises driving, increasing air pollution, carbon emissions and road deaths, wider societal costs which far outweigh any taxes on motoring. The cost of driving to society is around double the cost of fuel per mile.[52] The subsidies enjoyed by motoring could more usefully go towards active transport options that create health.

## Sustainable changes

Taxing carbon is the most effective way to start addressing the health and environmental impacts of climate change.[53] Our current economic system will stop polluting only when the cost of causing pollution is more than the cost of dealing with it. A solution to this failure of the market was proposed a century ago by the economist Arthur Pigou. A Pigouvian tax on activities generating negative externalities balances their cost to society, while a Pigouvian subsidy rewards activity generating wider benefit. Carbon taxes are a form of Pigouvian tax, attempting to price in the wider damage of our fossil fuel dependency.

Gross Domestic Product (GDP) is still considered the main measure of a country's economic activity. Metrics that value only what is priced miss the wider impacts of the economy. GDP records total economic activity, counted either as output, income or expenditure. GDP is not linked to happiness,[54] and is better at measuring the welfare of capitalism than the welfare of people.

Plenty of alternatives to GDP have been proposed which better reflect the wellbeing impacts of economic activity. The Genuine Progress Indicator (GPI) includes negative effects such as crime and damage to the environment within GDP, making a closer proxy for social economics. The Happy Planet Index combines wellbeing, life expectancy and equality, divided by ecological footprint.[55] The Better Life Index is derived from measures of housing, income, jobs, education, environment, health, life satisfaction, work-life balance, safety, community and civic engagement.[56] Other metrics include the Social Progress Index and the Index of Sustainable Economic Welfare.

The reliance on infinite growth within modern monetary practice is unsustainable on a finite planet. Growth requires resource use, resources that are increasingly scarce. Degrowth reorientates us towards a healthier, more equitable and more sustainable society.[57]

## How to talk about change

Talking about change helps to create it. The most effective way to frame actions is to ensure they align with positive emotions and core values, such as fairness, across both income divides and our responsibilities to other generations.[58] The language of climate catastrophe may convey urgency, but paradoxically may lead to a degree of fatalism in response. Similarly, medicalising inequality makes it far harder to solve.[59]

Framing provides the basis for interpreting information, integrating this with the pictures in our heads.[60] News stories are often framed as portraits, but introducing context gives instead a landscape view. Framing happens on different levels, one being our core values, such as fairness and reciprocity. Frames that resonate with shared values engage people. This is the stable base from which to address issues, and from there explore specifics. Policy detail needs to be built on core values.

Refuting a dominant framing can actually reinforce it, so changing the framing may be a more effective way of communicating an alternative. Referring to tax in terms of tax justice, for instance, evokes more responsive aspects of social identity.

Choice architecture refers to the effects on decision-making from the way choices are presented. This is used to direct consumer behaviour in stores which are designed to discombobulate and overwhelm shoppers to become less rational, acting instead on impulse (Gruen effect). Making the healthy option the default one is a powerful 'health by stealth' technique. Encouraging active travel, better nutrition and other health-promoting choices can be incentivised. Doing this at the local level engages community spirit and identification, raising social capital.

Subsidiarity means decisions should be taken as locally as necessary, encouraging accountability, and that values identified represent those of the community. Demonstrating effectiveness and following the evidence base should be at the heart of informed decision making. Supporting alternative provision helps to reclaim power from organisations. Cooperative methods to engage with transactions reduces corporate power, which avoids extraction of wealth and keeps investment in communities.[61]

## Open data

Ensuring change is sustainable requires processes to be transparent. Data sharing allows scrutiny, feedback and support, and the default position should be that data are shared, opening up a variety of potential uses. Healthcare data represent an incredibly rich hoard of information about demographics, treatments and outcomes to quantify risks and the effectiveness of interventions, but these should be available to all. The care.data scandal around previous attempts to commodify health data showed how public trust is eroded when personal data are sold to commercial interests.[62]

Health data are so detailed that identification of individuals becomes straightforward despite attempts to protect against this. Pseudonymisation of data is relied upon to hide identities for research, but even just two data points such as age and postcode narrow possibilities to a very small number of people, making it trivial to breach this level of security, especially by cross-referencing with other datasets.

The Goldacre review[63] looks at how NHS data can best be used to improve health while protecting patient confidentiality. The panoply of sources and complexity of data control make it hard for researchers to access data. Trusted research environments (TRE) host patient data as well as the code to process these data, allowing reproducibility. Ensuring data are made openly available should be embedded within public contracts. Automated access through application programming interfaces (APIs) allows wider utility of data and cross-pollination with other projects.

Spreadsheets are widely used within NHS analytics but provide no audit trail when curating data, making these data less reliable. Methods of processing data are robust if different analyses show the same results, and replicable if the same method gives the same results across different groups. Python and R are more mature and transparent open source tools for data analytics, with active user groups supporting use of these within healthcare analytics.[64, 65]

Open source refers to wider structures that are made available to others at no cost, freely sharable as long as no one tries to restrict rights. CC BY-XX copyleft licences allow use and sharing, with options around commercial use and redistribution. These licences share by default, ensuring that everything from software to designs for printable parts are available to use and develop. Sites such as github provide hosting and version control, allowing code to be used across multiple projects.

Open source software rivals and often outperforms proprietary operating systems. Code that is free to all and improvable by all allows better optimisation built on collaboration. This lets open source operating systems such as Linux run efficiently on older and slower hardware, reducing costs and waste from upgrades.

## Universal basic services

The large number of low-paid jobs with little job security threatens living standards for many.[66] One solution is a living stipend. This funds everyone to a basic standard, beyond which one can earn more by working. This supports without reinforcing the benefits trap, whereby receipt of benefits is conditional on proving unfitness to work. The need to show symptoms to access help with subsistence drives much low-value healthcare, at a higher cost than more direct support. In the recognition that moving to more helpful ways to ensure a basic standard of living for all is also cheaper, paying a universal basic income (UBI) is an effective way to support people and grow a local economy. Wider career choices arise from UBI, which makes it easier to escape for those at risk of abuse both at home and in the workplace.[67]

UBI may reinforce a market-based, 'individualist solution to a shared problem'.[68] Universal basic services (UBS) apply the same principles across a community, describing collectively generated, openly available services to meet basic needs. Including transport helps to decarbonise travel. UBS improves living standards and boosts jobs that aid the transition to a low-carbon economy.[69] These jobs are less reliant on financial markets, so are more resilient to recession. Pooling risk is the most effective way to create a safety net that covers needing external help.[70]

## Circular economy

Extractive systems bleed communities. Siphoning money into offshore accounts does not benefit a locality, but money spent in a local shop does. Money re-spent locally brings the same economic benefits to local trade as new money entering an area.

Counting money spent locally helps evidence decisions by showing the benefits of a circular economy. This requires focusing on the microeconomy to measure transactions and follow the flow of money. Money spent in a local economy can stay within that location or leak out. The LM3 local multiplier[71] counts how much money has been spent locally after three transactions (Table 10.1). Comparing the sum of all transactions to the original sum spent gives a ratio, which shows how value is cumulative during its journey through the economy. Shopping locally, preferring independent providers

*Table 10.1* LM3 local multiplier

| | |
|---|---|
| Original sum | £1,000 |
| if 75% of that spent locally | £750 |
| if 75% of that spent locally | £490 |
| | |
| Total local spend after 3 cycles | £2,190 |
| LM3 local multiplier ratio | £2,190 / £1,000 = 2.19 |

and cooperatives keeps money circulating locally and encourages a more diverse economy to thrive.

Corporate control, outsourced services and lack of diversity in economic output all contribute to money leaving a local economy. A more diverse range of smaller producers supports local production, reduces transport needs and increases resilience. Maintaining a distinct regional character encourages tourism and helps promote place identification.[72] The use of physical cash for transactions also promotes local spending rather than online purchases.

Alternative financial systems are another way to support local economies. These actively resist extractive systems by ensuring wealth circulates locally. Local exchange trading schemes (LETS) use alternative currencies to tally the exchange of goods and services. Interest is not chargeable, and trading retains value in the local economy. Time banks are another way to exchange services, swapping time which encourages reciprocity and local connections. Time banks build community capacity, improve self-esteem and confidence and increase prospects for employment.[73]

While LETS and time banked accrue to individuals, mutual credit is a means of exchange between networks of traders. Mutual credit schemes do not lead to inflation or hoarding, which reduces the risk of overconsumption, but instead return economic systems to communities.[74]

Transition towns address some of the changes needed to achieve sustainability by better coordination.[75] These recognise the primacy of communities and the future-proof structure they represent. Smaller communities derive a sense of cohesion while being responsive, although the natural footprint for each community will vary considerably according to geography, culture and other factors. Transition towns emphasise values that recognise the importance of connectedness; third places serving slow food, using local, seasonal produce, helps to maintain the identification and heritage of a locality.

Making changes requires engagement, which needs knowledge, motivation and the ability to act. The relationship between our thoughts and behaviours is not linear, meaning that change in one can happen without change in the other.[76]

Translating attitude into behaviour can be beset by the dragons of inaction,[77] the cognitive biases and other excuses we make or inherit for not making the changes we need to. Skewed perceptions of risk, sunk costs holding back changes and our various preconceptions and narratives all influence our behaviour.

Real change is not only possible but happening in communities across the world. Better connectedness lets us organise and make the case for change.

## Notes

Links and additional resources for this chapter can be found at www.communityhealth. uk/10-sustainable-policy

1  Turnpenny A, Hussein S. Migrant home care workers in the UK: a scoping review of outcomes and sustainability and implications in the context of Brexit. *J Int Migr Integr*. 2022;23(1):23–42. doi:10.1007/s12134-021-00807-3.
2  Tanner, Will, O'Shaughnessy, James, Krasniqi, Fjolla, Blagden, James. *The State of Our Social Fabric: Measuring the Changing Nature of Community over Time*

*and Geography*. Onward; 2020. https://www.ukonward.com/wp-content/uploads/2020/09/The-State-of-our-Social-Fabric.pdf

3 Office for Budget Responsibility. *Economic and Fiscal Outlook*. UK Government; 2022. https://obr.uk/download/economic-and-fiscal-outlook-march-2022/

4 'I think the people in this country have had enough of experts…from organisations with acronyms saying that they know what is best and getting it consistently wrong'. Michael Gove, Sky News, 3 June 2016. https://fullfact.org/blog/2016/sep/has-public-really-had-enough-experts/

5 Launer J. Medical activism. *Postgrad Med J*. 2021;97(1151):611–612. doi:10.1136/postgradmedj-2021-140809.

6 Palmer PJ. A new professional: the aims of education revisited. *Change Mag High Learn*. 2007;39(6):6–13. doi:10.3200/CHNG.39.6.6-13.

7 Hart E, Kuijpers G, Laverack G, Scheele F. The process leading to physician activism for sustainable change. *Sustainability*. 2021;13(18):10003. doi:10.3390/su131810003.

8 Myers TA, Nisbet MC, Maibach EW, Leiserowitz AA. A public health frame arouses hopeful emotions about climate change. *Clim Change*. 2012;113(3–4):1105–1112. doi:10.1007/s10584-012-0513-6.

9 Chapman, Jonathan. Democracy, redistribution, and inequality: evidence from the English poor law. Published online September 8, 2020. https://jnchapman.com/assets/pdf/poorlaw.pdf

10 Beveridge W. Beveridge report on voluntary action. *Mon Labor Rev*. 1949;68(4). http://www.jstor.org/stable/41831774

11 Jay, Douglas. *The Socialist Case*. Faber and Faber; 1937.

12 Brodie JM. Reforming social justice in neoliberal times. *Stud Soc Justice*. 2007;1(2):93–107. doi:10.26522/ssj.v1i2.972.

13 Coote, Anna, Penny, Joe. *The Wrong Medicine: A Review of the Impacts of NHS Reforms in England*. New Economics Foundation; 2014. https://neweconomics.org/2014/11/the-wrong-medicine/

14 Fotaki, Marianna. *What Market-Based Patient Choice Can't Do for the NHS: The Theory and Evidence of How Choice Works in Health Care*. Centre for Health and the Public Interest; 2014. https://chpi.org.uk/papers/analyses/market-based-patient-choice-cant-nhs-theory-evidence-choice-works-health-care/

15 Lent, Adam, Pollard, Grace, Studdert, Jessica. *A Community-Powered NHS: Making Prevention a Reality*. New Local; 2022. https://www.newlocal.org.uk/publications/community-powered-nhs/

16 Thatcher, Margaret. Interview for Woman's Own ('no such thing as society'). September 23, 1987. https://www.margaretthatcher.org/document/106689

17 Blair, Tony. Speech to Women's Institute. Women's Institute conference; June 7, 2000; Wembley, London. https://www.theguardian.com/politics/2000/jun/08/uk.labour2

18 Lupton R. What is neighbourhood renewal policy for? *People Place Policy Online*. 2013;7(2):66–72. doi:10.3351/ppp.0007.0002.0003.

19 Barr B, Bambra C, Whitehead M. The impact of NHS resource allocation policy on health inequalities in England 2001–11: longitudinal ecological study. *BMJ*. 2014;348(may27 6):g3231–g3231. doi:10.1136/bmj.g3231.

20 Kruger D. *Levelling up Our Communities: Proposals for a New Social Covenant*; 2020. https://www.dannykruger.org.uk/sites/www.dannykruger.org.uk/files/2020-09/Kruger%202.0%20Levelling%20Up%20Our%20Communities.pdf

21 Ibid.

22 Puddle, Jake, Rolfe, Heather. *Building Stronger Communities in Post-Pandemic Britain*. All Party Parliamentary Group on Social Integration; 2021. https://www.britishfuture.org/wp-content/uploads/2021/10/Building-stronger-communities.APPG-Social-Integration.pdf

23 CILIP. *Public Libraries: The Case for Support*. Department of Health and Social Care; 2019. https://www.cilip.org.uk/news/news.asp?id=599345

24  87% of towns benefitting from funding had Conservative MPs. Walker P, Allegretti A. Sunak's £1 bn of 'town deals' will nearly all go to Tory constituencies. *The Guardian*. https://www.theguardian.com/uk-news/2021/mar/03/sunaks-1bn-of-town-deals-will-nearly-all-go-to-tory-constituencies. Published March 3, 2021.

25  Davey F, McGowan V, Birch J, et al. Levelling up health: a practical, evidence-based framework for reducing health inequalities. *Public Health Pract*. Published online September 2022:100322. doi:10.1016/j.puhip.2022.100322.

26  'Robin Hood's redistributive army is missing when and where it is most needed'. Lindert PH. Three centuries of inequality in Britain and America. In: Atkinson, AB, Bourguignon, François, eds. *Handbook of Income Distribution*. Vol 1. Elsevier; 2000:167–216. doi:10.1016/S1574-0056(00)80006-8.

27  Wang Z, Jetten J, Steffens NK. Restless in an unequal world: economic inequality fuels the desire for wealth and status. *Pers Soc Psychol Bull*. Published online April 3, 2022:014616722210837. doi:10.1177/01461672221083747.

28  Iacobucci G. 'Levelling up' plan needs more funding and a focus on health inequalities, say experts. *BMJ*. Published online February 4, 2022:o303. doi:10.1136/bmj.o303.

29  Tudor Hart J. *The Political Economy of Health Care: A Clinical Perspective*. The Policy Press; 2006.

30  Hope D, Limberg J. The economic consequences of major tax cuts for the rich. *Socio-Econ Rev*. 2022;20(2):539–559. doi:10.1093/ser/mwab061.

31  Lena HF, London B. The political and economic determinants of health outcomes: a cross-national analysis. *Int J Health Serv*. 1993;23(3):585–602. doi:10.2190/EQUY-ACG8-X59F-AE99.

32  Page A. Suicide and political regime in New South Wales and Australia during the 20th century. *J Epidemiol Community Health*. 2002;56(10):766–772. doi:10.1136/jech.56.10.766.

33  d'Este R, Harvey A. The unintended consequences of welfare reforms: universal credit, financial insecurity, and crime. *J Law Econ Organ*. Published online July 9, 2022. doi:10.1093/jleo/ewac009.

34  Walsh D, Dundas R, McCartney G, Gibson M, Seaman R. Bearing the burden of austerity: how do changing mortality rates in the UK compare between men and women? *J Epidemiol Community Health*. Published online October 4, 2022:jech-2022-219645. doi:10.1136/jech-2022-219645.

35  Hardman I. *Why We Get the Wrong Politicians*. Atlantic Books; 2019.

36  Macfadyen, Peter. *Flatpack Democracy 2.0*. eco-logic books; 2020.

37  Bale, Tim, Cheung, Aron, Cowley, Philip, Menon, Anand, Wager, Alan. *Mind the Values Gap: The Social and Economic Values of MPs, Party Members and Voters*. The UK in a Changing Europe; 2020:19. https://ukandeu.ac.uk/wp-content/uploads/2020/06/Mind-the-values-gap.pdf

38  Dyer C. Covid-19: Government's use of VIP lane for awarding PPE contracts was unlawful, says judge. *BMJ*. Published online January 13, 2022:o96. doi:10.1136/bmj.o96.

39  Durkheim, Émile. *Suicide: A Study in Sociology*. Routledge; 1897.

40  Teymoori A, Bastian B, Jetten J. Towards a psychological analysis of anomie. *Polit Psychol*. 2017;38(6):1009–1023. doi:10.1111/pops.12377.

41  Lorenzoni I, Nicholson-Cole S, Whitmarsh L. Barriers perceived to engaging with climate change among the UK public and their policy implications. *Glob Environ Change*. 2007;17(3–4):445–459. doi:10.1016/j.gloenvcha.2007.01.004.

42  Brulle RJ. Institutionalizing delay: foundation funding and the creation of U.S. climate change counter-movement organizations. *Clim Change*. 2014;122(4):681–694. doi:10.1007/s10584-013-1018-7.

43  Hall S. Exxon knew about climate change almost 40 years ago. Scientific American. Published October 26, 2015. https://www.scientificamerican.com/article/exxon-knew-about-climate-change-almost-40-years-ago/

44 Garrett RK. Echo chambers online?: Politically motivated selective exposure among Internet news users. *J Comput-Mediat Commun.* 2009;14(2):265–285. doi:10.1111/j.1083-6101.2009.01440.x.

45 Swami V, Furnham A, Smyth N, Weis L, Lay A, Clow A. Putting the stress on conspiracy theories: Examining associations between psychological stress, anxiety, and belief in conspiracy theories. *Personal Individ Differ.* 2016;99:72–76. doi:10.1016/j.paid.2016.04.084.

46 Golec de Zavala A, Lantos D. Collective narcissism and its social consequences: the bad and the ugly. *Curr Dir Psychol Sci.* 2020;29(3):273–278. doi:10.1177/0963721420917703.

47 Leshem D. Retrospectives: What did the ancient Greeks mean by oikonomia? *J Econ Perspect.* 2016;30(1):225–238. doi:10.1257/jep.30.1.225.

48 The game of Monopoly, originally designed as a satire on the harms from land-grabbing, is based on accumulating unearned income to buckle the Lorenz curve into a right angle. In the game, everyone starts with the same amount of money. In real life, an initial seed is needed, a nidus for money to coalesce around, which is not available to those struggling with subsistence.

49 Smith, Adam. *An Inquiry into the Nature and Causes of the Wealth of Nations.* Strahan and Cadell; 1776.

50 Marx K. *Capital*, vol 1., 1981 standard ed. Penguin Books in association with New Left Review; 1867.

51 Tax Watch. *Equality before the Law? HMRC's Use of Criminal Prosecutions for Tax Fraud and Other Revenue Crimes. A Comparison with Benefits Fraud.* Tax Watch; 2021. https://www.taxwatchuk.org/tax_crime_vs_benefits_crime/

52 The societal cost of driving is £0.13/km, due to congestion, infrastructure provision, accidents, air quality, noise and greenhouse gases. Transport Appraisal and Strategic Modelling (TASM) Division. TAG data book v1.15. Published online July 2021. https://www.gov.uk/government/publications/tag-data-book

53 Watts N, Adger WN, Agnolucci P, et al. Health and climate change: policy responses to protect public health. *The Lancet.* 2015;386(10006):1861-1914. doi:10.1016/S0140-6736(15)60854-6.

54 O'Donnell, Gus, Deaton, Angus, Durand, Martine, Halpern, David, Layard, Richard. *Wellbeing and Policy.* Legatum Institute; 2014. https://li.com/reports/the-commission-on-wellbeing-and-policy/

55 Happy Planet Index. How happy is the planet? https://happyplanetindex.org/

56 Stefaner, Moritz, Rausch, Frank, Leist, Jonas, Paeschke, Marcus, Baur, Dominikus, Kekeritz, Timm. OECD Better Life Index. https://www.oecdbetterlifeindex.org/#/11111111111

57 Hickel J. *Less Is More: How Degrowth Will Save the World.* William Heinemann; 2020.

58 See note 3.

59 Lynch J. Reframing inequality? The health inequalities turn as a dangerous frame shift. *J Public Health.* 2017;39(4):653–660. doi:10.1093/pubmed/fdw140.

60 Dorfman L, Wallack L, Woodruff K. More than a message: framing public health advocacy to change corporate practices. *Health Educ Behav.* 2005;32(3):320–336. doi:10.1177/1090198105275046.

61 How to disengage from the corporate sector. https://www.noncorporate.org/

62 Godlee F. What can we salvage from care.data? *BMJ.* Published online July 14, 2016:i3907. doi:10.1136/bmj.i3907.

63 Goldacre, Ben, Morley, Jessica. *Better, Broader, Safer: Using Health Data for Research and Analysis.* Department of Health and Social Care; 2022. https://www.gov.uk/government/publications/better-broader-safer-using-health-data-for-research-and-analysis

64 Shenton CR. NHS Python Community Website. NHS Python Community Website. https://nhs-pycom.net/

65  NHS-R Community. Promoting the use of R in the NHS. https://nhsrcommunity. com/

66  Button, Daniel, Coote, Anna. *A Social Guarantee: The Case for Universal Services.* New Economics Foundation; 2021. https://neweconomics.org/2021/09/a-social-guarantee

67  Perkins G, Gilmore S, Guttormsen DSA, Taylor S. Analysing the impacts of Universal Basic Income in the changing world of work: challenges to the psychological contract and a future research agenda. *Hum Resour Manag J.* 2022;32(1):1– 18. doi:10.1111/1748-8583.12348.

68  Coote A, Percy A. *The Case for Universal Basic Services.* Polity; 2020.

69  See note 66.

70  See note 29.

71  Sacks J. *The Money Trail: Measuring Your Impact on the Local Economy Using LM3.* New Economics Foundation; 2002. https://neweconomics.org/uploads/ files/money-trial.pdf

72  Alexander M, Hamilton K. Recapturing place identification through community heritage marketing. *Eur J Mark.* 2016;50(7/8):1118–1136. doi:10.1108/EJM-05-2013-0235.

73  Singh, Sara. *The Evolution of Giving: An Exploration of Time Banking as a Community Development Instrument.* University of South Carolina; 2017. https:// timebanking.org/wp-content/uploads/2020/05/The-Evolution-of-Giving-An-Exploration-of-Time-Banking-as-a-Community-Development-Instrument.pdf

74  LowImpact.org. Mutual credit – an introduction. https://www.lowimpact.org/ categories/mutual-credit

75  Transition Network. Transition Towns. https://transitionnetwork.org/

76  See note 41.

77  The seven dragons of inaction: being unaware, ideological influences, comparisons, sunk costs, discredence, perceived risk and limited behaviour. Gifford R. The dragons of inaction: psychological barriers that limit climate change mitigation and adaptation. *Am Psychol.* 2011;66(4):290–302. doi:10.1037/a0023566

# 11 Developing community

Similar problems face communities across the world. Loneliness and social disconnection are common. The effects of inequality and climate injustice persist. Institutions professionalise responses, excluding citizens from involvement. Care systems are struggling because the economic and political systems they are based on are failing.[1]

Communities offer solutions to these problems. Supporting community development enhances capacity and competence. Engaging communities improves delivery of services, empowerment and social capital.[2] There is widespread agreement that developing community works; the Marmot review, the NHS Five Year Forward View, Public Health England and NICE have all called for place-based approaches to reduce health inequalities. These top-down calls for bottom-up approaches recognise the value of true asset-based development. Community mobilisation builds social capital, making us better able to withstand future crises.[3]

The direction of travel may be clear, but this still needs to translate into actual action. Individual participation comes when the barriers to involvement are lowered. Volunteers take part when 'offers of neighbourly service'[4] are easy to fulfil. Volunteers bring a rich and diverse mix of expertise, including group organisational skills. Understanding one's own skill set makes it easier to find an effective place to act from. Structures that empower people cultivate horizontal rather than vertical ties, as flatter hierarchies and bridging relationships allow more innovation. Teams that have the autonomy to solve their own issues spread power and create resilience.

## Promoting community

Statutory services are able to support communities directly.[5] The highest cost in care is staffing, salaries which enter the local economy. Services have significant buying power, which can be used to support smaller businesses by procuring goods and services locally. Spending supports neighbourhoods when considered as an investment in the local economy. Healthcare expenditure, rather than being a cost burden, generates four times the gross value of that investment in the local economy.[6]

DOI: 10.4324/9781003391784-12

Services can help in other ways. Professionals have useful skills and contacts, while health premises are also local assets. Health facilities often have space to host meetings, embedding these services into the local community. Staff working in health and care are trusted and well placed to understand the needs of patients.

Primary care networks offer a real chance to ensure investment is truly aimed at improving health locally. The new PCN additional roles offer ways to interface effectively with the VCS, both as outreach and a conduit back into health services. VCS representation is a crucial part of this.

## Community models

Desire lines are paths worn into the ground by people taking shortcuts, perfect examples of user-led design. Good design recognises and adapts, supporting but not controlling. Models of community that reflect the autonomy and diversity of citizen power celebrate the shortcuts, the local knowledge and flexibility to adapt to circumstances.

Services set up for the convenience of practitioners can instead be recentred around the needs of the community. Radical approaches develop capability rather than managing need, recognising the resources already present and creating possibilities.[7] Identifying community assets makes different forms of wealth visible.

Alternative funding models can better serve community needs. These include community shares, unique to co-operatives; perpetual bonds, in which money invested is not redeemable but pays interest forever; credit unions, which match investors and borrowers; and community foundations, which raise and spend funds locally.[8] The funding spectrum ranges from traditional models seeking pure financial return to philanthropic ones focused on impacts. Between these poles are various models to balance return and outcomes, which may be framed in terms of corporate or social responsibility. New models of exchange support a new economy.[9]

Community wealth building (the Preston model) uses wealth that is already present, the buying power of local authorities, to ensure money stays circulating within the area. A real living wage for staff and procurement based on social value keeps investment local and democratises the economy.

Community land trusts (CLT) are local non-profit organisations who purchase land for affordable housing that truly meets local needs. The CLT keeps the freehold and can lease or sell buildings, with the option to buy properties back in the future to keep them affordable.

Citizen science is another way to involve residents. A collaborative framework for collecting data informs participatory research and taps into local knowledge, but vested interests still need to be guarded against.[10]

These are all forms of *commoning*, the collaborative sharing of resources within a system of governance. This becomes an open-source, community-based way of looking after our resources equitably. Clear boundaries, local rules, participatory decision-making, and monitoring protect the commons, together with a way to enforce decisions when needed.[11]

*Good neighbour schemes* are an excellent example of practical community cohesion. A network of local volunteers with an organisational hub offers help when needed, whether giving lifts, running errands or other forms of support. These are services provided by the community, rather than located within the community.[12] These schemes are based on generalised reciprocity, helping by facilitating mutual support networks. Good neighbour schemes mobilise local residents to support each other.

Transport is a large part of the need, especially in rural areas. Good public transport allows people with dementia and disability to stay in rural communities. Sharing private forms of transport is part of this, reducing emissions and connecting people.

*Compassionate communities* grew from the recognition that professional services have reduced the role of communities in caring for people at home. More people want to die at home than do so, but lack of availability of care services means that admissions to hospital or hospice are common at the end of life. Empowering neighbours and friends to help forms two circles of care: an inner circle close to the patient providing physical care and emotional support and an outer circle contributing practical support.[13]

The Compassionate Frome project in Somerset expanded local social prescribing, and showed that developing a stronger sense of community has reduced health care use and improved outcomes. Frome showed a reduction in healthcare cost, with a 14 per cent decrease in unplanned hospital admissions at a time when admissions from the rest of Somerset increased by nearly 30 per cent.[14] Fleetwood similarly showed a reduction in emergency department attendances after adopting a health creation approach, involving residents to set up a community choir, gardening and support groups.[15]

The Frome project found four things were needed:

- mapping of existing community resources to compile a service directory
- formation of a network of willing volunteers, known as Community Connectors, offering support to those in need and guiding them to appropriate sources of help identified in the service directory
- formation of groups requested by members of the community to meet newly identified needs
- the creation of one-to-one support relationships through liaison with Health Connectors

Direct access to support, without the need of an expert or a prescription, is a key part of the success. Statutory services remain accessible but community-based resources are better placed to listen and respond to local need.

## Asset-based community development

Asset-based community development recognises and builds on assets that are already present. The aim is for citizens to reclaim activity, done by rather than done to.[16]

- By: done by us for us (asset based)
- With: nothing for us without us (co-production)
- For: everything done is done for us, without us (charity model)
- To: everything done is done to us, without us (medical model)

Three sets of building blocks are available: personal assets, collective assets and potential assets, which are those originating from outside the community.[17] Community assets are made up of stories, exchanges, neighbourhood places and the contributions of residents, associations and local institutions.[18]

Community assets are gifts of neighbours to each other. These can be gifts of the head, sharing information and wisdom; gifts of the heart, the emotional connections that generate care; gifts of the hands, practical, hands-on support; and gifts of conscience, the shared attitudes that create our sense of cohesion.[19]

## Asset mapping

Creating a map of local assets helps to understand and share what is already available in our communities. If there are gaps, why? What mechanisms would best stimulate capacity? If funding is available, where is it needed most?

Prioritising need has traditionally been the preserve of local councils, using Joint Strategic Needs Assessments (JSNA) to create a list of gaps. These reports collate and explore local statistics around health need, reporting to council Health and Wellbeing Boards (HWB). Risk factors, holes in services and outliers are identified, forming an official representation of the locality based on deficits. These 'maps of misery' represent a view of the community that inverts the perspective of people living there.[20]

Deficit mapping leads to 'categorical, divided, specialised, limited, technical, deficiency focused proposals'.[21] Accentuating deficits helps to make the case for funding, but viewing things through this negative lens makes it harder to create solutions. Plotting community assets instead enables 'treasure mapping', starting with what is strong rather than what is wrong. Directories of services make these maps available to all.

## Representation

The strength and resilience of community organisations comes from their diversity. Groups range from local branches of large national organisations with central funding and communications to tiny groups run on the enthusiasm of a handful of people. Such diversity gives an evolutionary advantage in difficult times, but this range also makes true representation complicated to achieve.

Representation of groups within wider decisions about provision is important but rarely resourced. Smaller groups have fewer people to share out attending meetings and so are less likely to be represented. A supportive infrastructure for community organisations provides an interface to engage with statutory bodies on behalf of groups.

Much of the inefficiency in running a VCS organisation comes from the time wasted in the endless search for funds. The predilection for short-term seed funding without help with ongoing costs makes it hard for groups to plan. Short-term contracts lead to job uncertainty and make retention of staff harder. Finding project money takes valuable time, which is far better spent on the activity the group exists to do. The role of coordinating funding could be taken on by an organisation representing groups and engaging with funders.

Match funding, in which central investment is predicated on locally con-tributed resources, has advantages as a funding model. Local involvement establishes local assets, and ensures that those ideas with genuine support are more likely to succeed. The resources offered for match funding need not be financial, as time or donations in kind can be used, engagement which justi-fies investment from others. Valuing time as much as financial input allows lower-income communities to compete successfully. Using peer groups to assess competing bids adds legitimacy to selection.

Citizen juries and assemblies are ways to involve people in policy, both at local and wider levels. The terms are sometimes used interchangeably, but juries have fewer people (one or two dozen) while assemblies should have enough people to be representative of the population served. Citizens work-ing together consider evidence provided by expert witnesses to create an informed recommendation. Without the pressure of seeking re-election, rep-resentatives are able to plan for the longer term.

Participatory budgets are decided by citizens, who recommend how public money should be spent. This process trusts residents to participate in deci-sion-making and to allocate real funding towards locally agreed priorities. 'Fugitive coproduction' is a collaboration of citizens and staff who do what is needed without asking permission.[22]

Many of these ideas are straightforward to implement, but are resisted by local political structures reluctant to share power. It is possible to break out of the traditional party system in local politics, but playing the party game may be necessary to achieve this. Flatpack Democracy describes how a group of independent councillors took over an ossified and unrepresentative coun-cil, and in the process reinvigorated representative democracy.[23] One of the most important functions was to open up council proceedings to allow a more diverse range of opinions and representation.

## Participation

How and where do we have the discussions needed to take these forward? Many of the exchanges that influence our social norms now take place on social media, the formats of which encourage superficial and polarised exchanges. Physical meetings remain the most productive forum for inter-actions. Third places already host discussions which reinforce or chal-lenge our norms and behaviours. More formally, the village or town hall has long been the place for debate. If this can also function remotely, it increases resilience. COVID-19 showed how behaviour change can occur quickly, but a social mandate is needed to ensure such behaviours persist.

Ensuring appropriate location, time and process is important, but also rec-ognising when and why people choose *not* to participate.[24] Accessible places to meet maximise participation. A warm welcome from someone greeting participants puts people at ease. Name badges and introductions are a quick way to open up the opportunity for connections.

Making change happen can be slow and frustrating. Sometimes reading the minutes and turning up to the meetings is the way to enable change, some-times it is in cultivating connections, or in the choices we make. Much of the change is individual: recognising institutional assumptions; when to step back; when to step up.

## Leadership

A good leader is someone who likes people, is a good listener, makes friends easily, builds trust easily, talks well, helps people believe in themselves, lets others take the credit, works hard, does not get discouraged too often, has a sense of their own identity, asks questions, is open to new ideas, is flexible, honest, self-disciplined, mature, courageous, sets limits, has vision and has a sense of humour.[25]

Leadership is not an individual task, but something that permeates through an organisation. Cascading procedures from the top down disempowers teams and loses the strengths of working together. Leadership, teamwork, communication, system design and learning and feedback are the crucial skills for complex situations.[26]

---

### Box 11.1   Developing a community

Some examples of community development follow. These are from Ross-on-Wye; similar groups, activities and connections are happen-ing in every town and neighbourhood, generating health and powering communities. Innovation and participation are everywhere, when we look.

The market town of Ross-on-Wye sits on a meander of the River Wye in Herefordshire, just on the English side of the Welsh border. Ross is celebrated as the birthplace of tourism, visitors travelling the Wye to admire the picturesque scenes. The town has a culture of philanthropy, and previous benefactors are still prominently remembered.

There is a huge amount of community activity. Ross Men's Shed does great work around the town maintaining and repairing assets such as benches. The community garden provides greenspace, food, company and a third place for meeting others and hosting activities. Hope Support provides valuable peer-led support for young people facing a family crisis. Ross has one of the first Meeting Centres for dementia in the country, which was the first to be set up directly by the community. Charity shops raise funds while giving clothes, toys, media and books a new lease of life. The walking and Equinox festivals, parkrun and sports clubs and groups make activity and wellbeing accessible.

## Ross CDT

Ross-on-Wye Community Development Trust (CDT) was born out of the need for an infrastructure to support and promote community development. This had been identified in the Neighbourhood Development Plan, and also by the town's mental health steering group, which had been looking at ways to develop social prescribing and address loneliness in the town. Local organisations found it useful to meet with each other, sharing information and addressing problems common to the groups. The most pressing need identified was low-level support for those who were struggling, with outreach to those most at risk. One nearby village employs a community support coordinator paid for by the parish to look out for people in the village who may be at risk.

The CDT was formed to support community groups with advice and information, to connect volunteers to groups and to be an interface with statutory providers such as health services and the council. Community Catalysts provided support and advice as the CDT was forming and the town council was supportive. Of the possible structures, a charitable incorporated organisation (CIO) met the needs of the CDT most flexibly. This limits liability for trustees and gives the abilities of a corporate body without being subject to the regulations for companies.

The first project for the CDT was to set up a Good Neighbour Scheme. This was aimed at increasing connectedness in the community to reduce loneliness and isolation. Neighbourhood teams cover each part of town, supporting people with shopping, pet care and other tasks. Volunteers know their patch, have had training and are able to support and signpost towards appropriate help. This was the original vision, but the pandemic led to volunteers organised more by function than place, teams based around offering a particular function. From these teams, a role can be matched to a local volunteer. Making teams skills-based rather than place-based increases the range offered and should reduce role strain.

The CDT keeps members informed of opportunities and developments. A regular newsletter highlighting local community activity goes through every letterbox in town. Training events cover topics such as safeguarding and mental health first aid. Other projects include free DBS checks for local volunteer groups, a community oximeter library, signposting to debt advice and helpline support for those who are not digitally enabled to access online services. Work is ongoing to make Ross a dementia-friendly town, building on the support already in place.

Project Clover was a joint partnership between Ross CDT and other providers. Based on the five ways to wellbeing approach, the project offered a number of free activities for people in Ross and the surrounding villages. A website provides a menu of options, with links based on options: Create, Learn, Outdoors, Volunteer, Exercise, Relate. Priority for bookings went initially to social prescribers, before being opened up to all. Taster sessions were introduced to reduce the chance of participants dropping out and thus a space being lost. The website continues as an ongoing resource.[27]

Connections with others benefit health. Helping to establish these connections is a worthwhile way to enable health. Signposting and individual support to access activities are effective ways to regain the health improvements that associational life brings. Whether through a link worker or a neighbour, ensuring our communities are welcoming generates connections and social capital.

Groups enhance ties to others, which increases our options and resilience. Spending time in greenspace, playing and being active is strongly health-creating. Growing, preparing and eating local food is good for bodies and minds. Taking ownership of our infrastructure makes for a more inclusive and neurotolerant society. Creating the environment for activity and active travel enables health.

Support to develop community capacity and competence benefits health and wellbeing, both directly and through wider economic and environmental effects. Community development improves our health, our relationships, our environment and the wider society around us.

## Tips

Start small, with achievable aims, and build from there (Jim Diers)[28]

Start where people are. This means respecting their concept of what a community is, which may not be geographical[29]

An organiser should never do for people what they can do for themselves (Saul Alinsky)[30]

Good leaders give us a sense of who we are, not just who they are (Si Kahn)[31]

Support while stepping back (Cormac Russell)[32]

If you see someone struggling, ask them to help you (Camerados)

Revolution, one experiment at a time (Kate Raworth)

Tell a new story (Hilary Cottam)[33]

Don't have a meeting when you can have a party (Jim Diers)[34]

### Checklist: key issues in participation processes

- Situation assessment – interests, stakeholders, barriers[35]
- Self-assessment – what is feasible?
- Clarifying purpose, values and vision – what is the aim?
- Roles and responsibilities
- Increasing commitment, understanding non-involvement
- Communication
- Developing criteria for what matters
- Negotiation to agree on what and how
- Accessing resources
- Developing skills/capacities
- Generating options creative solutions
- Making decisions
- Developing organisational structures
- Managing structure skills and resources
- Evaluating progress – how is success judged?

### Checklist: community empowerment

- Community participation[36]
- Assessment of issues
- Leadership
- Structures
- Mobilising resources
- Links with others
- Critical awareness, asking 'why?'
- Community control
- Equitable relationships with outside agencies

## Notes

Links and additional resources for this chapter can be found at www.communityhealth. uk/11-developing-community

1 Cottam, Hilary. *Welfare 5.0: Why We Need a Social Revolution and How to Make It Happen.* UCL Institute for Innovation and Public Purpose; 2020. https://www. ucl.ac.uk/bartlett/public-purpose/wp2020-10

2 Milton B, Attree P, French B, Povall S, Whitehead M, Popay J. The impact of community engagement on health and social outcomes: a systematic review. *Community Dev J.* 2012;47(3):316–334. doi:10.1093/cdj/bsr043.

3 Costello A, Abbas M, Allen A, et al. Managing the health effects of climate change. *The Lancet.* 2009;373(9676):1693–1733. doi:10.1016/S0140-6736(09)60935-1.

4 Beveridge W. Beveridge report on voluntary action. *Mon Labor Rev.* 1949;68(4). http://www.jstor.org/stable/41831774

5 McKnight, John. *The Careless Society: Community and Its Counterfeits.* Basic Books; 1995.

6 Wood, Michael, Bosch, Ilse. *From Safety Net to Springboard: Putting Health at the Heart of Economic Growth.* NHS Confederation; 2022. www.nhsconfed.org/ publications/safety-net-springboard

7 Cottam H. *Radical Help: How We Can Remake the Relationships between Us and Revolutionise the Welfare State.* Virago; 2018.

8 Gregory, Dan. *Levelling the Land: Social Investment and "left behind" Places.* Local Trust; 2021. https://localtrust.org.uk/wp-content/uploads/2021/11/Levelling-the-land_November-2021.pdf

9 LowImpact.org. Sustainable living info, courses, products & services. https:// www.lowimpact.org/categories/main/economy

10 Kythreotis AP, Mantyka-Pringle C, Mercer TG, et al. Citizen social science for more integrative and effective climate action: a science-policy perspective. *Front Environ Sci.* 2019;7:10. doi:10.3389/fenvs.2019.00010.

11 Ison RL, Straw E. *The Hidden Power of Systems Thinking: Governance in a Climate Emergency.* Routledge; 2020.

12 Coxon, Kate, Smith, Teresa. *Good Neighbour Schemes in England: Community Support "in between" the Statutory and Voluntary Sectors.* Oxford Social Research Ltd; 2011.

13 Abel J, Kellehear A, Karapliagou A. Palliative care – the new essentials. *Ann Palliat Med.* 2018;7(S2):S3–S14. doi:10.21037/apm.2018.03.04.

14 Abel J, Kingston H, Scally A, et al. Reducing emergency hospital admissions: a population health complex intervention of an enhanced model of primary care and compassionate communities. *Br J Gen Pract.* 2018;68(676):e803–e810. doi:10.3399/bjgp18X699437.

15 Forrester V. My PCN: how healthier Fleetwood neighbourhood blazed a trail. Healthcare Leader. Published April 28, 2020. https://healthcareleadernews.com/ case-studies/my-pcn-how-healthier-fleetwood-neighbourhood-blazed-a-trail/

16 Russell C. *Rekindling Democracy: A Professional's Guide to Working in Citizen Space.* Cascade Books; 2020.

17 Blickem C, Dawson S, Kirk S, et al. What is asset-based community development and how might it improve the health of people with long-term conditions? A realist synthesis. *SAGE Open.* 2018;8(3):215824401878722. doi:10.1177/ 2158244018787223.

18 McKnight, John, Russell, Cormac. The four essential elements of an asset-based community development process: what is distinctive about an asset-based community development process? Published online September 2018. https://www. nurturedevelopment.org/wp-content/uploads/2018/09/4_Essential_Elements_of_ ABCD_Process.pdf

19 Russell C, McKnight J. *The Connected Community: Discovering the Health, Wealth, and Power of Neighborhoods*. Berrett-Koehler Publishers Inc; 2022.

20 Abel, Julian. Survival of the Kindest Podcast: Angela Fell, the function of a neighbourhood.https://compassionate-communitiesuk.co.uk/podcast/34-survival-of-the-kindest-angela-fell-the-function-of-a-neighbourhood/

21 Kretzmann, John, McKnight, John. *Building Communities from the inside out: A Path towards Finding and Mobilizing a Community's Assets*. abcd Institute; 1993.

22 Stewart E. Fugitive coproduction: conceptualising informal community practices in Scotland's hospitals. *Soc Policy Adm*. 2021;55(7):1310-1324. doi:10.1111/spol.12727.

23 Macfadyen, Peter. *Flatpack Democracy 2.0*. eco-logic books; 2020.

24 Cornwall A. Unpacking "participation": models, meanings and practices. *Community Dev J*. 2008;43(3):269–283. doi:10.1093/cdj/bsn010.

25 Kahn, Si. *Organizing, a Guide for Grassroots Leaders*. NASW Press; 1992.

26 Al-Azri NH. Antifragility amid the covid-19 crisis: making healthcare systems thrive through generic organisational skills. *Sultan Qaboos Univ Med J SQUMJ*. 2020;20(3):241. doi:10.18295/squmj.2020.20.03.001.

27 Ross CDT. CLOVER: Creative, Leisure, Outdoor & Volunteering Opportunities in the Ross-on-Wye area. https://clover-hr9.org.uk/

28 Diers, Jim. *Neighbor Power*. University of Washington Press; 2004.

29 See note 18.

30 Alinsky SD. *Rules for Radicals: A Practical Primer for Realistic Radicals*. Vintage Books; 1989.

31 See note 25.

32 Agdal, Rita, Midtgård, Helen, Russell, Cormac. *Asset-Based Community Development - How to Get Started*. Western Norway University of Applied Sciences; 2019. https://www.abundantcommunity.com/files/Asset-Based_Community_Development_ABCD_-_A_Booklet_for_Residents.pdf

33 Cottam, Hilary. Blog: Radical health. Published June 22, 2022. https://www.hilarycottam.com/radical-health/

34 See note 28.

35 Wilcox D. *The Guide to Effective Participation*. Partnership Books; 1994.

36 Laverack G. *Public Health: Power, Empowerment and Professional Practice*. Palgrave; 2005.

# Further resources

Links and additional resources can be found at www.communityhealth.uk/further-resources

## Communities

Canter, David. *The Psychology of Place*. Architectural Press; 1977.

Keller, Suzanne. The American dream of community: an unfinished agenda. *Sociol Forum*. 1988; 3(2): 167–183. doi:10.1007/BF01115289.

Parsfield, Matthew, David Morris, Manjit Bola, et al. *Community Capital: The Value of Connected Communities*. RSA Action and Research Centre; 2015. www.thersa.org/globalassets/pdfs/reports/rsaj3718-connected-communities-report_web.pdf

Putnam, Robert D. *Bowling Alone: The Collapse and Revival of American Community*. Simon & Schuster; 2001. ISBN 978-0-74320-304-3.

## Inequality

Richard, Wilkinson, Kate Pickett. *The Spirit Level: Why Equality Is Better for Everyone*. Penguin; 2009. ISBN 978-0-14103-236-8.

## ACEs and trauma

Van Der Kolk, Bessel. *The Body Keeps the Score*. Penguin; 2014. ISBN 978-014197-861-1.

## Healthcare

Davies, James. *Sedated: How Modern Capitalism Created our Mental Health Crisis*. Atlantic Books; 2021. ISBN: 978-1-78649-987-5.

Dowrick, Christopher. *Beyond Depression: A New Approach to Understanding and Management*. Oxford University Press; 2004. ISBN 978-0-19852-632-2.

Hart, Julian Tudor. *The Political Economy of Health Care: A Clinical Perspective*. The Policy Press; 2006. ISBN 978-1-86134-808-1.

Illich, Ivan. *Medical Nemesis: The Expropriation of Health*. Calder & Boyars; 1974. ISBN 978-0-71452-993-6.

Kitwood, Tom, Kathleen Bredin. Towards a theory of dementia care: personhood and well-being. *Ageing Soc*. 1992; 12: 269–287. doi: 10.1017/s0144686x0000502x.

Kleinman, Arthur, Anne E Becker. "Sociosomatics": the contributions of anthropology to psychosomatic medicine. *Psychosom Med*. 1998; 60(4): 389–393. doi:10.1097/00006842-199807000-00001.

McKnight, John. *The Careless Society: Community and its Counterfeits*. BasicBooks; 1995. ISBN 978-0-46509-126-3.

Russell, Cormac. Does more medicine make us sicker? Ivan Illich revisited. *Gac Sanit.* 2019; 33(6): 579–583. doi:10.1016/j.gaceta.2018.11.006.

## Social prescribing

Bragg, Rachel, Gavin Atkins. *A review of nature-based interventions for mental health care*. Natural England Commissioned Reports, Number 204. 2016. http://publications.naturalengland.org.uk/publication/4513819616346112

Friedli, Lynne, Catherine Jackson, Hilary Abernethy, Jude Stansfield. *Social Prescribing for Mental Health – a Guide to Commissioning and Delivery*. CSIP North West Social Prescribing Development Project; 2008. https://citizen-network.org/library/social-prescribing-for-mental-health.html

Social Prescribing team, Personalised Care Group NHSe. *Social prescribing link workers: Reference guide for primary care networks – Technical Annex.* June 2020. www.england.nhs.uk/wp-content/uploads/2020/06/pcn-reference-guide-for-social-prescribing-technical-annex-june-20.pdf

## Social infrastructure

Department for Digital, Culture, Media and Sport. *Rapid Evidence Review of Community Initiatives*. UK Government; 2022. www.gov.uk/government/publications/rapid-evidence-review-of-community-initiatives

Klinenberg, Eric. *Palaces for the People: How to Build a More Equal and United Society*. Crown; 2018. ISBN 978-1-78470-751-4.

Roe, Jenny, Layla McCay. *Restorative Cities: Urban Design for Mental Health and Wellbeing*. Bloomsbury Visual Arts; 2021. ISBN 978-1-35011-288-9.

South, Jane. *A Guide to Community-Centred Approaches for Health and Wellbeing*. Public Health England; 2015. PHE publications gateway number: 2014711 www.gov.uk/government/publications/health-and-wellbeing-a-guide-to-community-centred-approaches

Swift, Carolyn, Gloria Levin. Empowerment: an emerging mental health technology. *J Primary Prevent*. 1987; 8: 71–94. https://doi.org/10.1007/BF01695019

Wilcox, David. *The Guide to Effective Participation*. Brighton: Partnership Books; 1994. ISBN 978-1-87029-800-1.

Yarker, Sophie. *Creating Spaces for an Ageing Society: The Role of Critical Social Infrastructure*. Emerald Publishing; 2022. ISBN 978-1-83982-739-6.

## Planetary health

Costello, Anthony, Mustafa Abbas, Adriana Allen, et al. Managing the health effects of climate change. *The Lancet*. 2009; 373(9676): 1693–1733. doi:10.1016/S0140-6736(09)60935-1.

Hallegatte, Stephane, Adrien Vogt-Schilb, Mook Bangalore, Julie Rozenberg. Unbreakable: Building the Resilience of the Poor in the Face of Natural Disasters. In *Climate Change and Development Series*. World Bank; 2017. doi:10.1596/978-1-4648-1003-9; https://elibrary.worldbank.org/action/showCitFormats?doi=10.1596%2F978-1-4648-1003-9_ov

Hulme, Mike. *Why We Disagree About Climate Change: Understanding Controversy, Inaction and Opportunity*. Cambridge University Press; 2009. ISBN 978-0-52172-732-7.

IPCC. Summary for Policymakers. In Masson-Delmotte, V., P. Zhai, A. Pirani, S.L. Connors, C. Péan, S. Berger, N. Caud, Y. Chen, L. Goldfarb, M.I. Gomis, M. Huang, K. Leitzell, E. Lonnoy, J.B.R. Matthews, T.K. Maycock, T. Waterfield, O. Yelekçi, R. Yu, and B. Zhou (eds.). *Climate Change 2021: The Physical Science Basis. Contribution of Working Group I to the Sixth Assessment Report of the Intergovernmental Panel on Climate Change.* Cambridge University Press; 2021. https://www.ipcc.ch/report/ar6/wg1/chapter/summary-for-policymakers/

Raworth, Kate. *Doughnut Economics: Seven Ways to Think Like a 21st-Century Economist.* Random House; 2017. ISBN 978-1-84794-139-8.

Rockström, Johan, Will Steffen, Kevin J. Noone, et al. Planetary boundaries: exploring the safe operating space for humanity. *Ecol Soc.* 2009; 14(2): 32. www.ecologyandsociety.org/vol14/iss2/art32/

Watts, Nick, W Neil Adger, Paolo Agnolucci, et al. Health and climate change: policy responses to protect public health. *Lancet.* 2015; 386(10006): 1861–1914. doi: 10.1016/S0140-6736(15)60854-6.

Webb, Jonathan, Lucy Stone, Luke Murphy, Jack Hunter. *The Climate Commons: How Communities Can Thrive in a Climate Changing World.* Institute for Public Policy Research; 2021. www.ippr.org/research/publications/the-climate-commons

### Sustainable policy

Coote, Anna, Andrew Percy. *The Case for Universal Basic Services.* Polity; 2020. ISBN: 978-1-50953-983-3.

Hickel, Jason. *Less Is More: How Degrowth Will Save the World.* William Heinemann; 2020. ISBN 978-1-786-091215.

Low Impact Co-operative. www.lowimpact.org

Macfadyen, Peter. *Flatpack Democracy 2.0.* Eco-logic Books; 2020. ISBN 978-1-899233-27-4.

The Turing Way Community. (2021). *The Turing Way: A Handbook for Reproducible, Ethical and Collaborative Research* (1.0.1). Zenodo. doi: 10.5281/zenodo.3233853.

### Community development

Abel, Julian. *Survival of the Kindest Podcast.* https://compassionate-communitiesuk.co.uk/podcasts/

Abel, Julian, Lindsay Clarke. *The Compassion Project: A Case for Hope and Humankindness from the Town That Beat Loneliness.* Aster; 2020. ISBN 978-1-78325-336-4.

Alinsky, Saul. *Rules for Radicals: A Practical Primer for Realistic Radicals.* Vintage Books; 1989. ISBN 978-0-67972-113-0.

Bagnall, Anne-Marie, Jane South, Salvatore Di Martino, et al. *Places, Spaces, People and Wellbeing: Full Review. A Systematic Review of Interventions to Boost Social Relations through Improvements in Community Infrastructure (Places and Spaces).* What works wellbeing; 2018. https://whatworkswellbeing.org/resources/places-spaces-people-and-wellbeing/

Cottam, Hilary. *Radical Help: How We Can Remake the Relationships between Us and Revolutionise the Welfare State.* Virago; 2018. ISBN 978-0-34900-909-4.

Kahn, Si. *Organizing, a Guide for Grassroots Leaders.* NASW Press; 1992. ISBN 978-0-87101-197-8.

Lent, Adam, Grace Pollard, Jessica Studdert. *A Community-Powered NHS: Making Prevention a Reality*. New Local; 2022. www.newlocal.org.uk/publications/community-powered-nhs/

McKnight, John, Peter Block. *The Abundant Community: Awakening the Power of Families and Neighborhoods*. Berrett-Koehler Publishers, Inc; 2012. ISBN 978-1-60994-081-2.

Russell, Cormac. *Rekindling Democracy: A Professional's Guide to Working in Citizen Space*. Cascade Books; 2020. ISBN 978-1-72525-363-6.

Russell, Cormac, John McKnight. *The Connected Community: Discovering the Health, Wealth, and Power of Neighborhoods*. Berrett-Koehler Publishers Inc; 2022. ISBN 978-1-52300-252-8.

# Acknowledgements

I am indebted to those who made this book better. Amrit Sachar, Dave Darby, Jade Woolley, Jane Roberts, Julia Kelly, Kit Byatt, Mark Waters, Matt Rose and Tonia Chester all helped me make sense of what I was trying to say. The mistakes are mine alone.

Thanks to Alice Rose, Ben Rose and Casey Ord for comments and suggestions, and Linda Dykes for her 'GP as universal sink plug' analogy.

So many people worked on the local projects described, but especially Anne Parsons, Anne-Marie Dossett, Brenda Read-Brown, Christine Price, Jane Mainey, Jane Roberts, Melvin Reynolds, Nigel Lane, Phil Shackell, Ruth Worgan, Tess Brooks and Tim Shelley. Philip Clayton and Richard Cook always supported the surgery as part of the wider community. Those who volunteer make their communities healthier and happier as a result.

Thanks to Henry, William and Tonia for their love and support.

# Glossary

**ACEs** adverse childhood experiences, potentially traumatic experiences in formative years

**Acuity** the severity of an illness

**Acute** short-term or of quick onset

**ADHD** attention deficit hyperactivity disorder

**Allostatic load** the physical results of chronic stress

**Anomie** a breakdown in norms leading to social disintegration

**APIs** application programming interfaces which automate access to data

**ARRS** additional roles reimbursement scheme, which funds newer roles within PCNs such as clinical pharmacists and first contact practitioners (*FCPs*)

**Atherosclerosis** plaque buildup inside arteries leading to heart disease and strokes

**Attention restoration theory** the propensity of nature to improve our ability to concentrate

**Barker hypothesis** poor nutrition in the womb sets up cardiovascular risk later in life

**BCF** better care fund, a pooled budget between the NHS and local authorities

**Biological determinism** the idea that human behaviour and outcomes are hereditary rather than influenced by our surroundings

**Biophilia** an innate link between humans and other life forms

**Blue prescribing** promoting activities for wellbeing on or around water

**Bonding ties** connections between people with similar characteristics

**Bridging ties** connections between people with different characteristics

**CAMHS** child and adolescent mental health services

**Cartesian dualism** Descartes' separation of body and mind

**CBT** cognitive behavioural therapy, talking therapy mainly provided within the *NHS* by *IAPT*

**CCG** clinical commissioning group, responsible for commissioning healthcare in an area

**CFCs** chlorofluorocarbons used as propellants in inhalers

**Choice architecture** structures influencing consumer choices

**Chrematistics**   the accumulation of money, maximising short term gains (see also *oikonomia*)

**Chronic**   ongoing

**Chronos**   linear time

**Circular economy**   limiting waste and emissions by sharing, reusing and recycling

**Citizen assemblies**   a group of citizens convened to discuss an issue

**Client media**   media supporting rather than challenging authority

**CLT**   community land trust, a non-profit organisation that holds land for community benefit

**Coenaesthesia**   awareness of inhabiting our bodies

**Coherence, sense of**   where the world is manageable, understandable and has meaning

**Collective narcissism**   a group belief of superiority to others

**Commission bias**   a tendency towards action even if it does not alter the outcome

**Commissioning**   translating need into provision of services

**Commoning**   collaborating to share a common resource

**Community identification**   the extent to which community members perceive they share the norms of the community

**Co-morbidity**   co-existing health conditions

**Compassionate community**   one that supports neighbours with care, often towards the end of life

**Competence**   the ability of communities to manage and solve problems of collective life

**Comprehensibility**   as part of *generalised resistance resources*, how understandable stimuli are

**Conservation medicine**   a medical field covering the health of humans, animals and ecosystems

**Copyleft**   the right to use, copy and share, typically software or digital resources

**Cortisol**   a hormone produced by the adrenal glands which regulates stress responses

**Countertransference**   the therapist's reaction to a patient

**CQC**   Care Quality Commission, health and social care regulator

**CRP**   C-reactive protein, a marker of inflammation in blood tests

**DALY**   a disability-adjusted life year of life lost

**Degrowth**   decoupling from a growth-based economy to transition to a more equitable and sustainable society

**Eco-anxiety**   worries about environmental catastrophe

**ED**   emergency department, also known as accident and emergency

**EMDR**   eye movement desensitisation and reprocessing, a form of psychological therapy for dealing with traumatic memories

**Emergent resilience**   response to chronic adversity

**Empowerment**   gaining autonomy and self-determination

**Epigenetics**   environmental triggers altering the expression of genes

**Eudaimonia**   a life well lived

**Exercise on prescription**   referral for exercise or physical activity

**FCP**   first contact practitioner, musculoskeletal specialists (usually physio-therapists) working in *primary care*

**FFP**   filtering face piece masks

**Five ways to wellbeing**   advice on staying healthy based on connecting, staying active, taking notice, learning and giving

**Flow**   the feeling of being absorbed completely in an activity

**Fugitive coproduction**   unauthorised collaboration between residents and staff

**GAD-7**   generalised anxiety disorder questionnaire

**Generalised resistance resources**   those that facilitate coping, in particular a sense of meaning

**Gini coefficient**   the difference between actual distribution of wealth and a fair share

**Glucose tolerance**   the ability to process glucose effectively, which is impaired in diabetes

**Good neighbour scheme**   local volunteers organised to support each other

**GP**   general practitioner, a generalist doctor working in primary care, sometimes known as family practitioner

**GPPAQ**   General Practice Physical Activity Questionnaire

**Green prescribing**   promoting activities in natural environments

**Greenspace**   community spaces with vegetation

**Group consulting**   consecutive individual consultations in a group setting

**Healthwatch**   local statutory organisations facilitating patient involvement in health and social care

**Hegemony**   domination or influence over others

**HEPA**   high-efficiency particulate air filters

**HFCs**   hydrofluorocarbons used as inhaler propellants

**Homophily**   attraction to those who share similar characteristics

**HWB**   Health and Wellbeing Boards, local authority forum comprising *NHS*, *public health* and local government involvement

**Hyperlocal**   pertaining to a very specific local area, smaller than local

**IAPT**   improving access to psychological therapies, the main *NHS* talking therapy provision

**ICB**   integrated care board, statutory organisation responsible for local provision of health services

**ICP**   integrated care partnership brings together *NHS*, local authority and other stakeholders

**ICS**   integrated care system, organisational partnership to meet health and care needs

**IMD**   index of multiple deprivation, a relative rank of deprivation by locality

**Impostor phenomenon**   an internalised belief of lacking the competence perceived by others

**Incorporation**   the maturation of the political self

**Isolation**   an objective lack of social contacts (see also *loneliness*)

**JSNA**   joint strategic needs assessment, an assessment of the health and wellbeing needs of a local area

**Just-world hypothesis**   a cognitive bias assuming that if something bad happens, it must have been deserved

**Kairos**   the opportune moment, a qualitative experience of time

**LETS**   local exchange trading scheme, a community based exchange of services using local currency

**Link worker**   see *social prescriber*

**Local authority**   local government organisation, such as County or District Council or Unitary Authority

**Local multiplier**   money re-spent in the local economy

**Locus of control**   the degree to which an individual feels in control over the things that affect their life

**Loneliness**   a subjective feeling of lacking companionship (see also *isolation*)

**Long Covid**   persisting symptoms following COVID-19 infection

**Lorenz curve**   a graphical representation of income inequality

**LSOA**   lower super output area, an organisational area of around 1,500 residents

**LTNs**   low traffic neighbourhoods, schemes minimising through-traffic in residential streets

**Manageability**   the availability of resources to help coping

**Matthew effect**   whereby the rich get richer and the poor get poorer

**MCC**   mortality cost of carbon, the increase in deaths per tonne of $CO_2$

**MDT**   multi disciplinary team

**MECC**   making every contact count, brief opportunistic health promotion

**MET**   metabolic equivalent of task, a measure of the energy expenditure of an activity

**Microbiome**   the bacteria sharing our bodies

**Microflow**   short duration purposeful action at the edge of awareness, such as doodling

**Minimal-impact resilience**   response to acute life event

**Morbidity**   ill but alive

**Mortality**   not alive

**MSOA**   middle super output area, organisational areas of between 5,000 and 15,000 residents

**MUS**   medically unexplained symptoms, or medically unexplored stories

**Mutual aid**   acts of solidarity among people coming together to meet a shared need or concern

**NEET**   not in employment, education or training, typically school leavers who disengage with societal activities

**NHS**   National Health Service, public healthcare provision in the UK which is free at the point of care

**Nosocomial**   hospital or healthcare acquired

**Oikonomia**   prudent household management (see also *chrematistics*)

**ONS**   Office for National Statistics

**Open source**   accessible designs which can be modified and shared

**Palma ratio**   measure of inequality comparing the top decile of earnings with the bottom four deciles

**PAM**   patient activation measures, assessment of confidence and ability to manage one's own health

**PAR**   participatory action research, enquiry into social change involving participants

**PCN**   primary care network, a group of local *GP* surgeries and other community providers

**PCT**   primary care trust, former organisation ensuring local health delivery (replaced by *CCGs*)

**Peer support**   help from people with similar health conditions

**Personal budgets**   money to fund a care plan

**PHQ-9**   patient health questionnaire looking at symptoms of depression

**Pigouvian**   taxation or subsidy to reflect externalised costs

**Place identification**   how residents define a place

**PLR**   public living rooms, shared spaces supported by the Camerados movement

**PPE**   personal protective equipment

**ppm**   parts per million

**Precariat**   a social class with insecure or unpredictable income

**Primary care**   generalist health care with direct access

**PROMs**   patient reported outcome measures

**Proxy markers**   biochemical or other parameters to measure disease rather than outcome data

**PTSD**   post-traumatic stress disorder

**Public health**   promoting health and preventing disease

**Public service mutuals**   previously public sector organisations which aim to have a positive social impact

**QALY**   a quality-adjusted life year gained

**Reasonable worst case scenario**   the worst plausible outcome to be planned for

**Resilience**   the ability to adapt to adversity; also, a way to pass responsibility onto the individual

**Robin Hood index**   measure of inequality reflecting the difference between actual share of income and a fair share

**Role strain**   the stress of fulfilling a role, especially where this increases over time

**SDOH**   social determinants of health, the social and economic circumstances that influence health

**Secondary care**   specialist care needing referral

**Self-efficacy**   belief in ability to manage a particular task

**Self-identity**   the story we tell about ourselves

**Sense of coherence**   things making sense cognitively and emotionally

**Sequelae**   the ongoing consequences of a disease

**Slacktivism**   online activity supporting political or social causes

**Social cost of carbon**   the societal cost of climate change per tonne of $CO_2$

**Social identity**   the story others would tell about us

**Social medicine**   improving health by addressing societal and economic determinants of health

**Social prescriber**   a non-clinical worker connecting patients with community sources of support (also known as a *link worker*)

**Social prescribing**   the use of non-medical sources of support

**Solastalgia**   distress caused by losses due to climate change

**SROI**   social return on investment, a way of measuring the social, environmental and financial impact of an intervention

**State capture**   policy influenced by private interests for their own advantage

**STP**   sustainability and transformation plan, commissioning footprint covering multiple PCNs

**Stress recovery theory**   the calming influence of nature

**Subsidiarity**   the principle that decisions should be taken at the most local level possible

**Surplus powerlessness**   an internalised belief that change cannot happen

**Sympathetic tone**   relative excess of the 'fight-or-flight' part of the nervous system that prepares us for emergencies

**Symptom blizzard**   numerous unrelated symptoms presented across multiple bodily systems

**Symptom shift**   relocation of symptoms elsewhere in the body, sometimes in response to normal investigations

**Telomeres**   cellular scaffolds supporting chromosomes, susceptible to the effects of stress

**Tertiary care**   specialised services usually within larger hospitals

**Third places**   social environments outside of the home or workplace

**Toxic stress**   chronic and damaging exposure to traumatic experiences

**Transactional analysis**   a modality of psychotherapy focusing on the interactions between parent, adult and child ego states

**Transference**   the unconscious redirection of feelings onto another

**Trauma informed communities**   widespread community understanding of the effects of trauma

**TRE**   trusted research environments, secure analytics platforms hosting health data

**Triple bottom line accounting**   accounting practices which include people and planet as well as prosperity

**u3a**   University of the Third Age, a nationwide network of learning groups aimed at older people

**VCS**   voluntary and community sector, non-statutory community based organisations and groups

**VCSE**   voluntary, community and social enterprise, see *VCS*

**VRUs**   vulnerable road users such as pedestrians and cyclists

**Weltschmerz**   'world-pain', distress at the state of the world

**WEMWBS**   Warwick-Edinburgh mental wellbeing scale

**WHO**   World Health Organisation

**Zoonotic**   disease transmissible from animals to humans

# Credits

Figure 1.1, reproduced with permission, from Canter D. *The Psychology of Place*.

Figures 3.1 and 3.2, reproduced with permission, from Kitwood T, Bredin K. Towards a Theory of Dementia Care: Personhood and Well-being. *Ageing Soc.* 1992;12(03):269-287.

Figure 3.6, reproduced with permission, from Donabedian A. *An Introduction to Quality Assurance in Health Care*, with thanks to Richard Youatt and Professor Varduhi Petrosyan.

Figure 6.1, parkrun finish time data kindly provided by Chrissie Wellington

Figure 9.1, adapted from *The Doughnut of social and planetary boundaries*, 2017 by Kate Raworth and Christian Guthier. CC-BY-SA 4.0. Raworth, K. (2017), *Doughnut Economics: seven ways to think like a 21st century economist*. London: Penguin Random House.

Figure 10.1, reproduced with permission, from Teymoori A, Bastian B, Jetten J. Towards a psychological analysis of anomie. *Polit Psychol.* 2017;38(6):1009-1023. doi:10.1111/pops.12377 (an error in the originally published image has been corrected)

# Index

Pages in *italics* refer to figures and **bold** refer to tables.